Depigmentation

Edited by Tae-Heung Kim

Published in London, United Kingdom

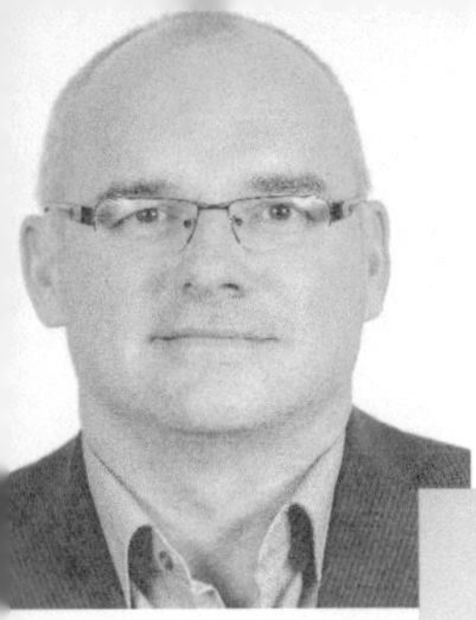
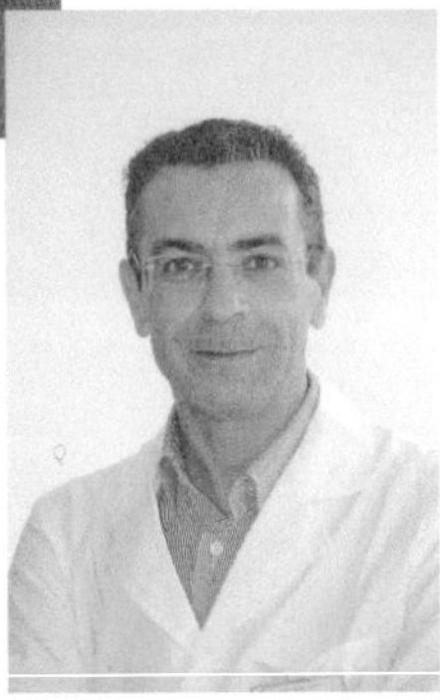
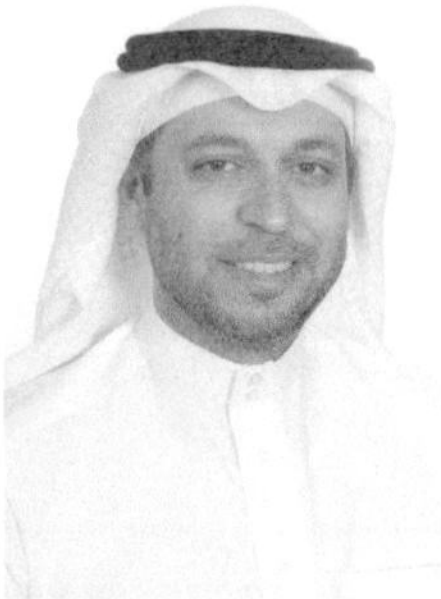
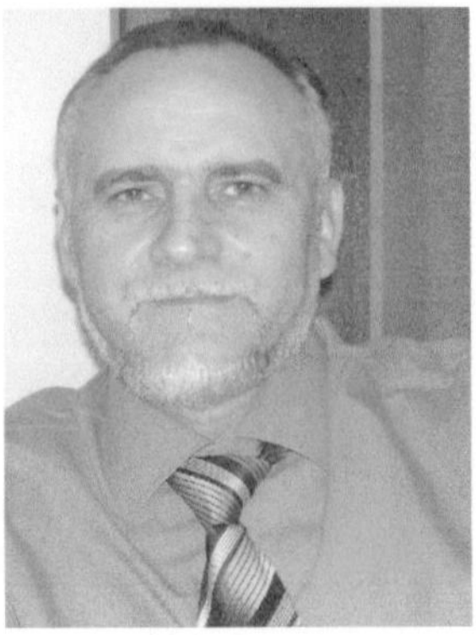
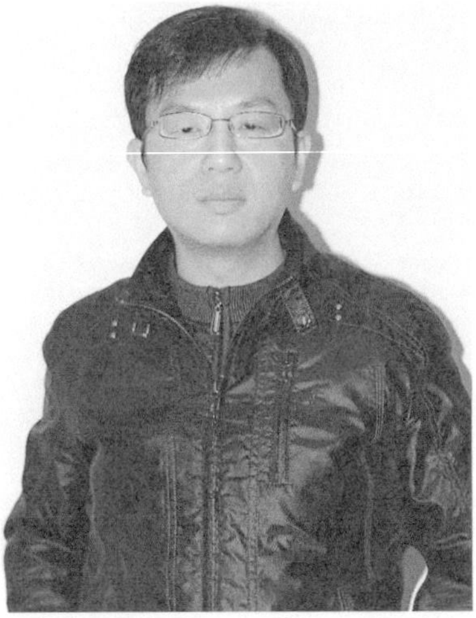
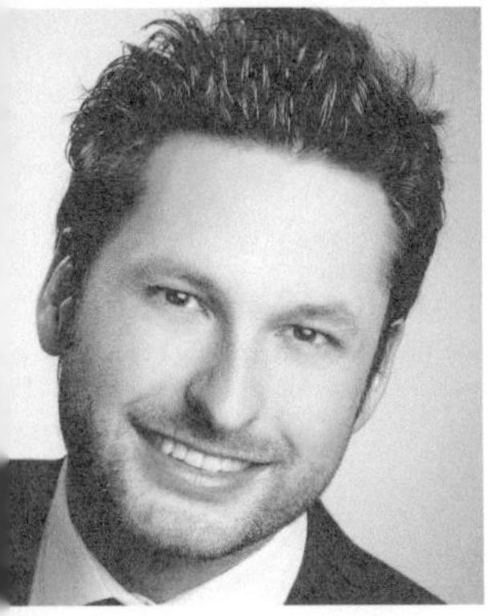
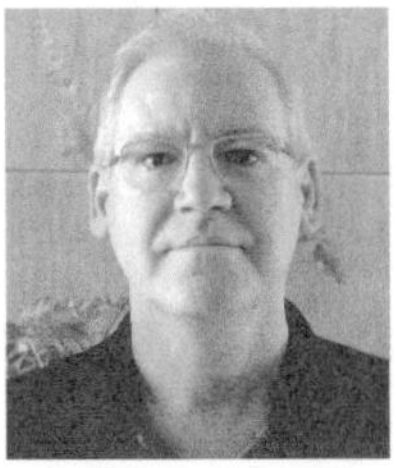

IntechOpen

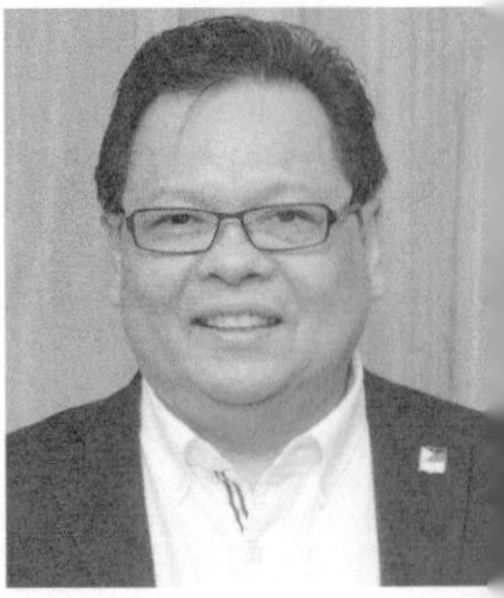
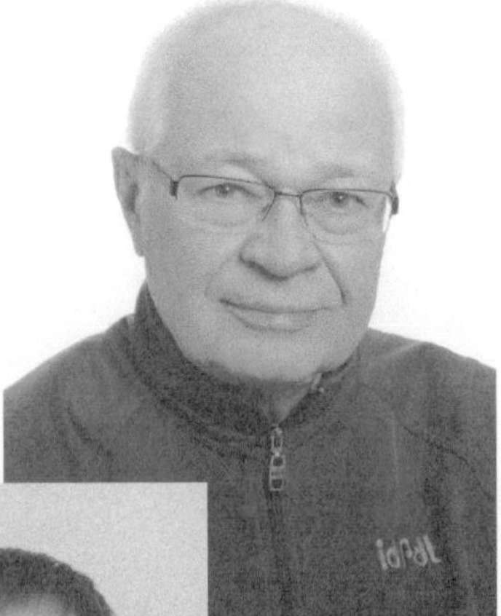
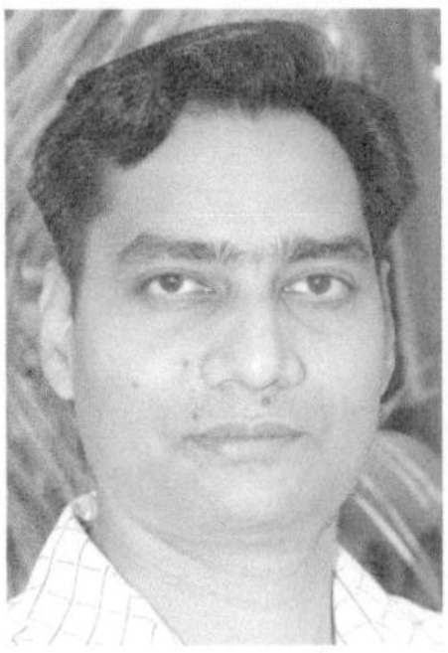
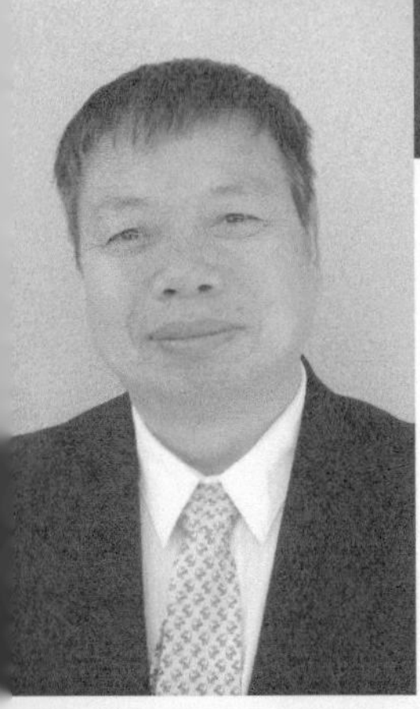
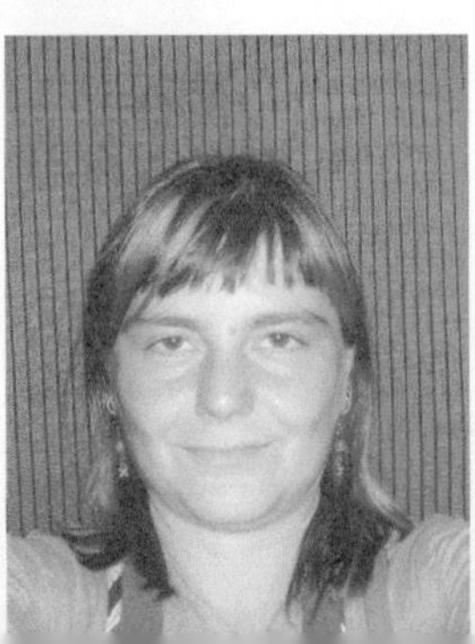
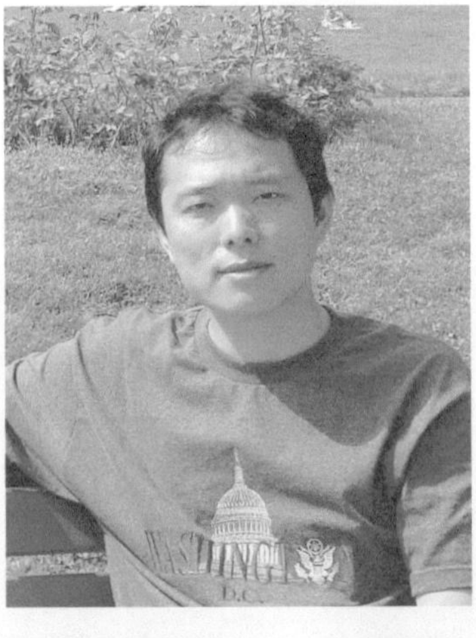

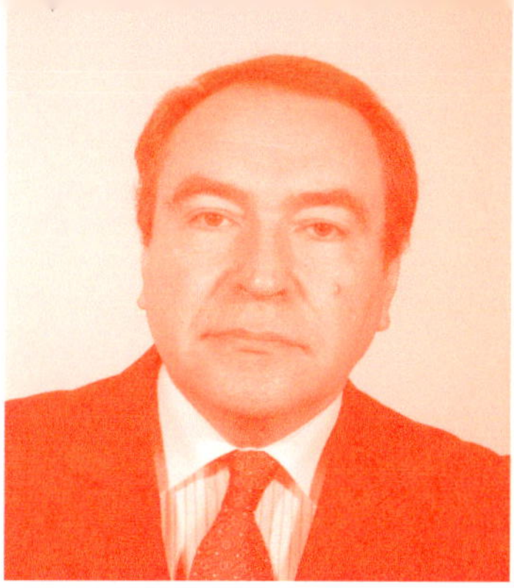
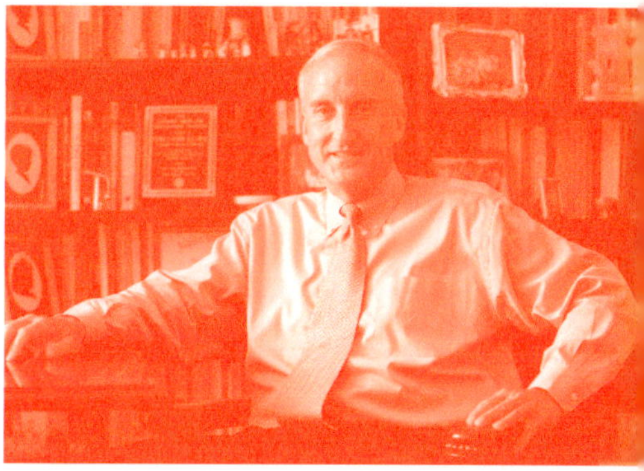
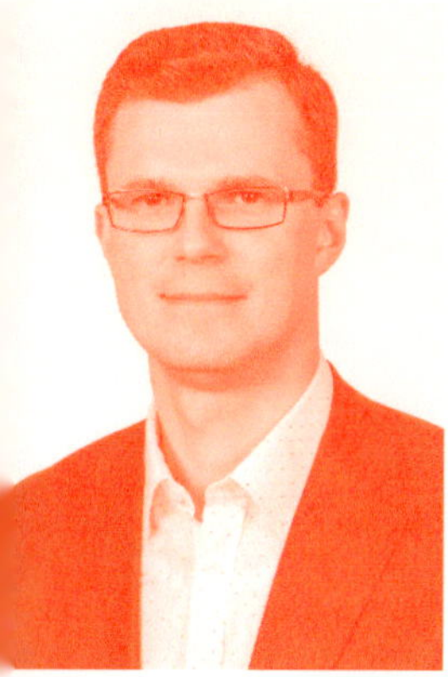
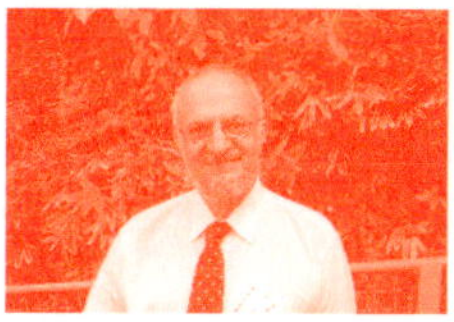
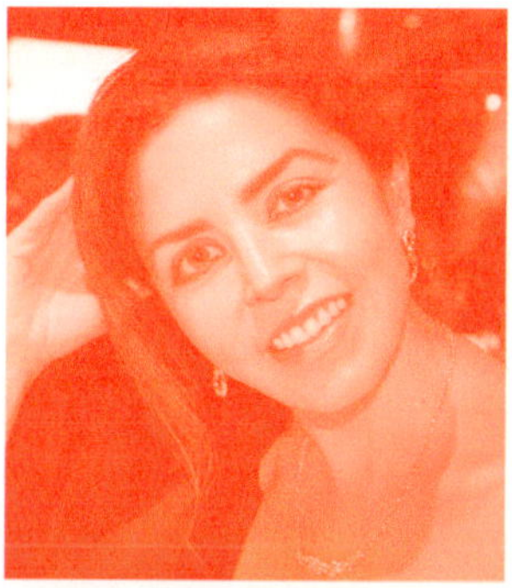

Supporting open minds since 2005

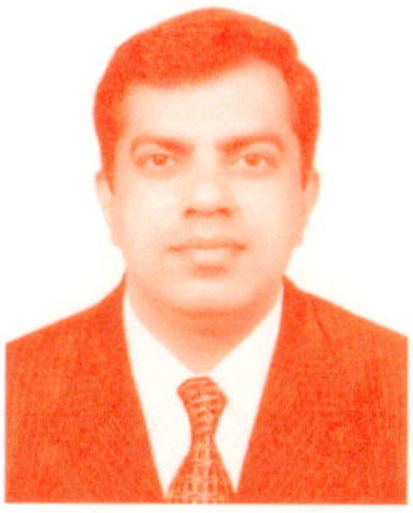
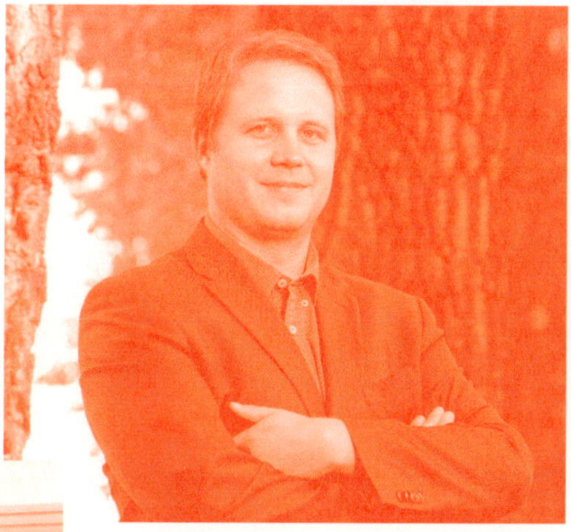
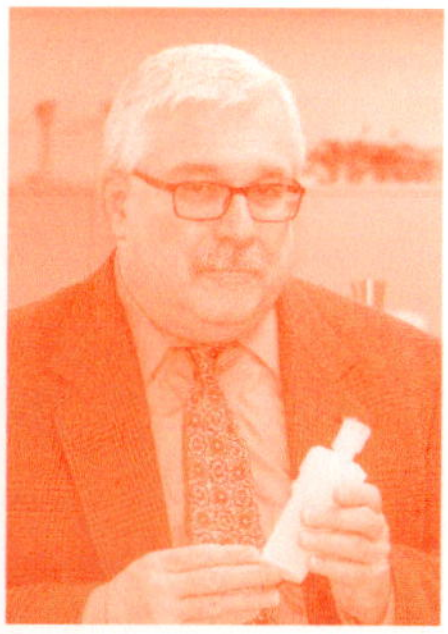
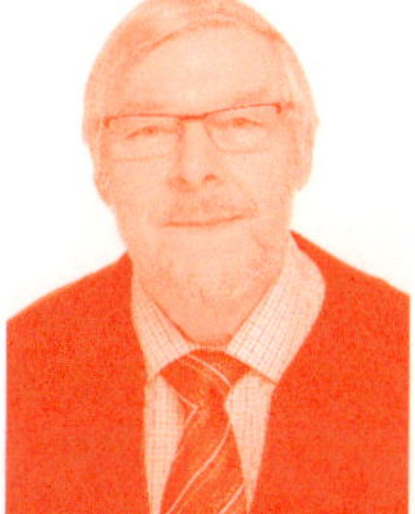
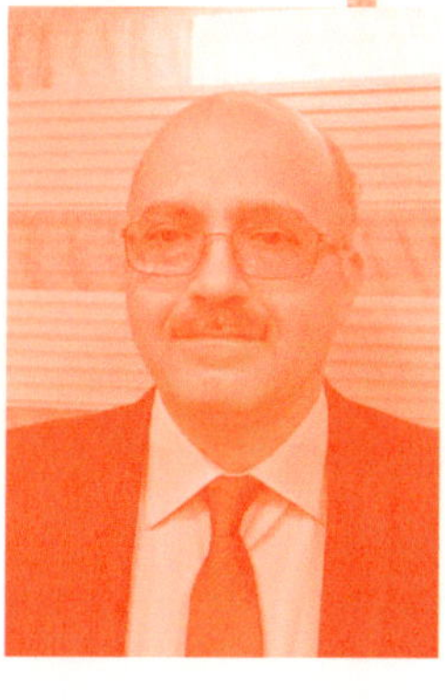
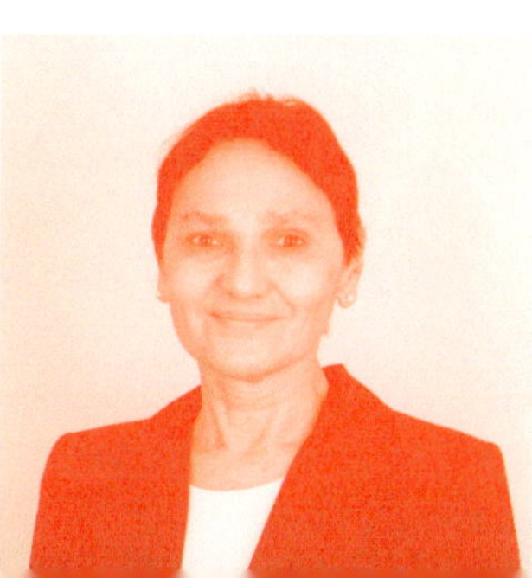
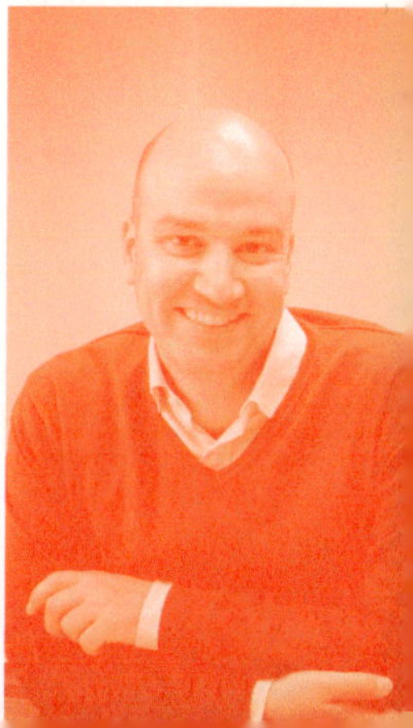

Depigmentation
http://dx.doi.org/10.5772/intechopen.73943
Edited by Tae-Heung Kim

Contributors
Amit Kumar Yadav, Işıl Kamberoğlu Turan, Panagiotis Tsikouras, Fotis Gasparos, Georgia Saradi, Xanthoula Anthoulaki, Theodora Deftereou, Anastasia Bothou, Anna Chalkidou, Dimitrios Tzeferakos, Eleftherios Chatzimichael, Georgios Iatrakis, Stefanos Zervoudis, Georgios Galazios, Sanjeev Mulekar, Madhulika Mhatre, Swapnil Mulekar, Naima Parveen, Sharique A. Ali, Ayesha S. Ali, Tae-Heung Kim

First published in London, United Kingdom, 2019 by IntechOpen
IntechOpen is the global imprint of INTECHOPEN LIMITED, registered in England and Wales, registration number: 11086078, 7th floor, 10 Lower Thames Street, London, EC3R 6AF, United Kingdom
Printed in Croatia

British Library Cataloguing-in-Publication Data
A catalogue record for this book is available from the British Library

Additional hard and PDF copies can be obtained from orders@intechopen.com

Depigmentation
Edited by Tae-Heung Kim
p. cm.
Print ISBN 978-1-83880-082-6
Online ISBN 978-1-83880-321-6
eBook (PDF) ISBN 978-1-83880-322-3

Meet the editor

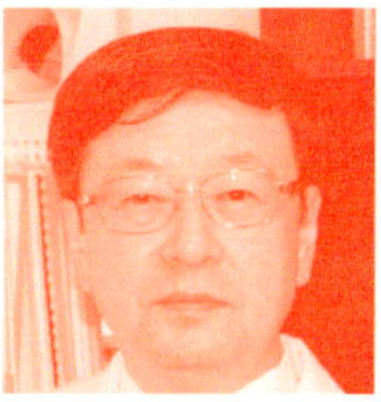

Dr. Tae-Heung Kim graduated from and acquired a doctoral degree (PhD) at Seoul National University College of Medicine. He completed an internship and dermatology residency at Seoul National University Hospital.
He moved to the Department of Dermatology, Gyeongsang National University, and was then promoted to Professor and Chairman of Dermatology. In 1996, he did a research sabbatical for two years at the Department of Immunology, University of Texas MD Anderson Cancer Center. In 2003, he started private practice as Director of the White-Line Skin Clinic and Research Center, Changwon, Kyungnam. He is an active member of many international and domestic societies, and was the President of the Korean Society for Vitiligo (2016–2018).

Contents

Preface

Depigmentation (lightening of the skin and mucosa) can be caused by local or systemic conditions, and there may be partial or complete loss of pigment. Depigmented patches have serious implications for pigmented skin. Depigmentation can also be a therapeutic goal for cosmetic treatment. In this book, we will focus on both sides of depigmentation; diseases of depigmentation and therapeutic depigmentation presented by global experts.

Dr. Kamberoğlu Turan summarized about the use of lasers in the treatment of vitiligo. This chapter includes the 308 nm excimer laser and supplementary use of fractional carbon dioxide or erbium-YAG laser for repigmentation treatment of vitiligo, and the Q-switched laser for the depigmentation of remaining normal skin.

Dr. Yadav presented interesting points on the histopathology and molecular pathology of vitiligo.

Depigmentation can also affect mucosal structures. Depigmentation of female genitalia can cause severe shame and it can also be a sign of malignancy. Prof. Tsikouras and colleagues have reviewed benign depigmentation disorders of the vulva and clinical management, and have included clear clinical photographs.

When a vitiligo patch is big, therapeutic depigmentation is an easier and more convenient way to help patients. Dr. Mulekar summarized depigmentation therapies in vitiligo.

Cosmeceutical depigmentation is a big market for investigators and cosmetic companies. Ms. Parveen and colleagues presented a very interesting paper about how depigmenting cosmeceuticals improve hyperpigmentation.

I appreciate the contributions from all of the authors for their excellent academic efforts.

I want to thank my family, Eun-Mee Kim (Gil), Na-Hyun and Keun-Woo who comfort my life. I always feel deep thanks to Prof. Ai-Young Lee and Seung-Kyung Hann, who worked on vitiligo as my colleague dermatologists and personal tutors for thirty years. And finally, I wish to thank all of the staff members of the White-Line Skin Clinic and patients of depigmentation diseases.

Tae-Heung Kim, MD, Ph.D.
White-Line Skin Clinic and Research Center,
Changwon,
Kyungnam,
Korea

Section 1

Diseases of Depigmentation

Chapter 1

Introductory Chapter: Depigmentation

Tae-Heung Kim

1. Introduction

Depigmentation, lightening of the skin and mucosa, can be caused by local or systemic conditions, and there may be partial or complete loss of pigment [1]. Although depigmented patches may not matter in Caucasians, it is very serious for pigmented skin [2]. Depigmentation can also be a therapeutic goal for cosmetic treatment. Many vitiligo patients, who received depigmentation treatment, experience paradoxical jealousy because of their clean white skin. To improve facial blemishes, many people spend their money for laser, chemical peel, and cosmeceutical [3, 4].

Depigmentation can occur hereditarily or acquiredly. Hereditary diseases if depigmentation includes following diseases (**Figure 1**) [3]. Oculocutaneous albinism consists of a group of genetic disorders characterized by diffuse pigmentary dilution due to a partial or total absence of melanin pigment within melanocytes of the skin and eyes. Piebaldism is an genetic disorder characterized by poliosis and congenital, stable, circumscribed areas of leukoderma due to an absence of melanocytes within involved sites. Waardenburg syndrome is a rare genetic disease characterized by various combinations of depigmentation of skin and irides, and congenital deafness. Hermansky–Pudlak syndrome is a rare genetic disease of depigmentation showing pigmentary dilution of the skin, hair, and eyes, and serious systemic manifestations including hematopoietic, immune, pulmonary, renal, and cardiac symptoms. Chédiak–Higashi syndrome is a rare genetic disorder showing features of oculocutaneous albinism, ocular symptoms, hematologic and neurologic manifestations. Tuberous sclerosis complex is an autosomal dominant disorder characterized by neuroligic disorders and skin findings including depigmented macules. Depigmentation along the lines of Blaschko reflects mosaicism characterized by a clone of skin cells with a decreased ability to make pigment. Hypomelanosis of Ito, linear nevoid hypopigmentation and nevus depigmentosus are considered to represent manifestations of cutaneous mosaicism.

Acquired diseases of depigmentation includes vitiligo, hypomelanosis secondary to cutaneous inflammation (postinflammatory hypopigmentation, pityriasis alba, sarcoidosis, hypopigmented mycosis fungoides, lupus erythematosus and lichen sclerosus et atrophicus), infectious hypomelanosis (tinea versicolor, leprosy, kala azar...), chemical or pharmacologic hypomelanosis (chemical leukoderma, hypomelanosis by strong steroid), hypomelanosis from physical agetnts (burn, laser, abrasion...), and miscellaneous (idiopathic guttate hypomelanosis, persistent macular hypomelanosis...) (**Figure 2**) [3].

Diseases of depigmentation can occur hereditarily or acquiredly. Hereditary diseases of depigmentation were reviewed excellently by Prof. Carrasquillo and colleagues. Albinism, piebaldism, white patches of tuberous sclerosis, Hermansky-Pudlak syndrome, Chédiak-Higashi syndorme, Waardenburg syndrome, and

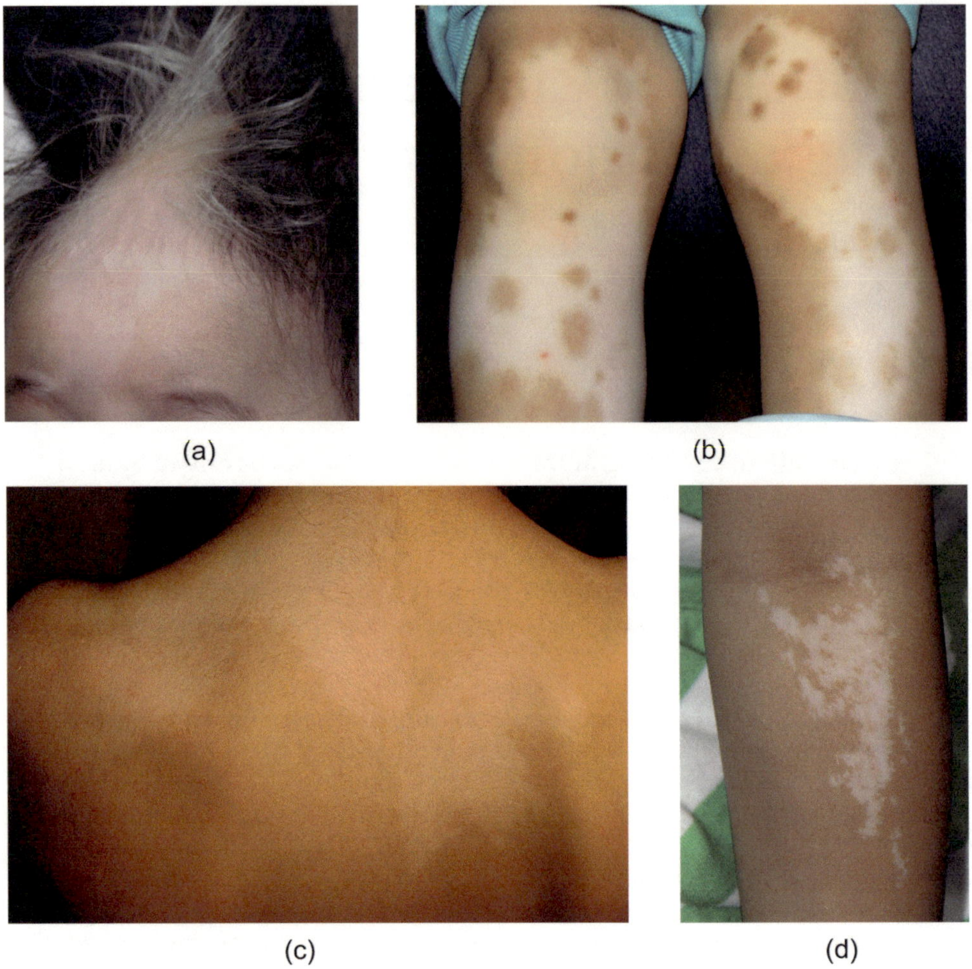

Figure 1.
Hereditary diseases of depigmentation. a. White forelock of piebaldism. b. Piebaldism affecting legs. c. Linear nevoid hypopigmentation. d. Nevus depigmentosus.

pigmentary mosaicism including hypomelanosis of Ito and nevus depigmentosus would be examples of them (**Figure 1**) [3].

Acquired diseases of depigmentation includes vitiligo, hypomelanosis secondary to cutaneous inflammation (postinflammatory hypopigmentation, pityriasis alba, sarcoidosis, hypopigmented mycosis fungoides, lupus erythematosus and lichen sclerosus et atrophicus), infectious hypomelanosis (tinea versicolor, leprosy, kala azar...), chemical or pharmacologic hypomelanosis (chemical leukoderma, hypomelanosis by strong steroid), hypomelanosis from physical agetnts (burn, laser, abrasion...), and miscellaneous (idiopathic guttate hypomelanosis, persistent macular hypomelanosis...) (**Figure 2**) [3].

Vitiligo is a common acquired disease of depigmentation, and afflicts and frightens so many patients. In vitiligo, melanocytes that produces melanin pigment of the skin are destroyed, and it can occur systemically to affect whole body or locally/segmentally affecting part of the body (**Figure 2a** and **b**) [3].

For the treatment of vitiligo, various lasers including 308 nm excimer laser are used successfully which has been used additionally with phototherapy and topical or systemic medications [5].

In patients with extensive vitiligo, depigmentation can be an easier and cosmetically more acceptable option. It includes various chemical and physical modalities.

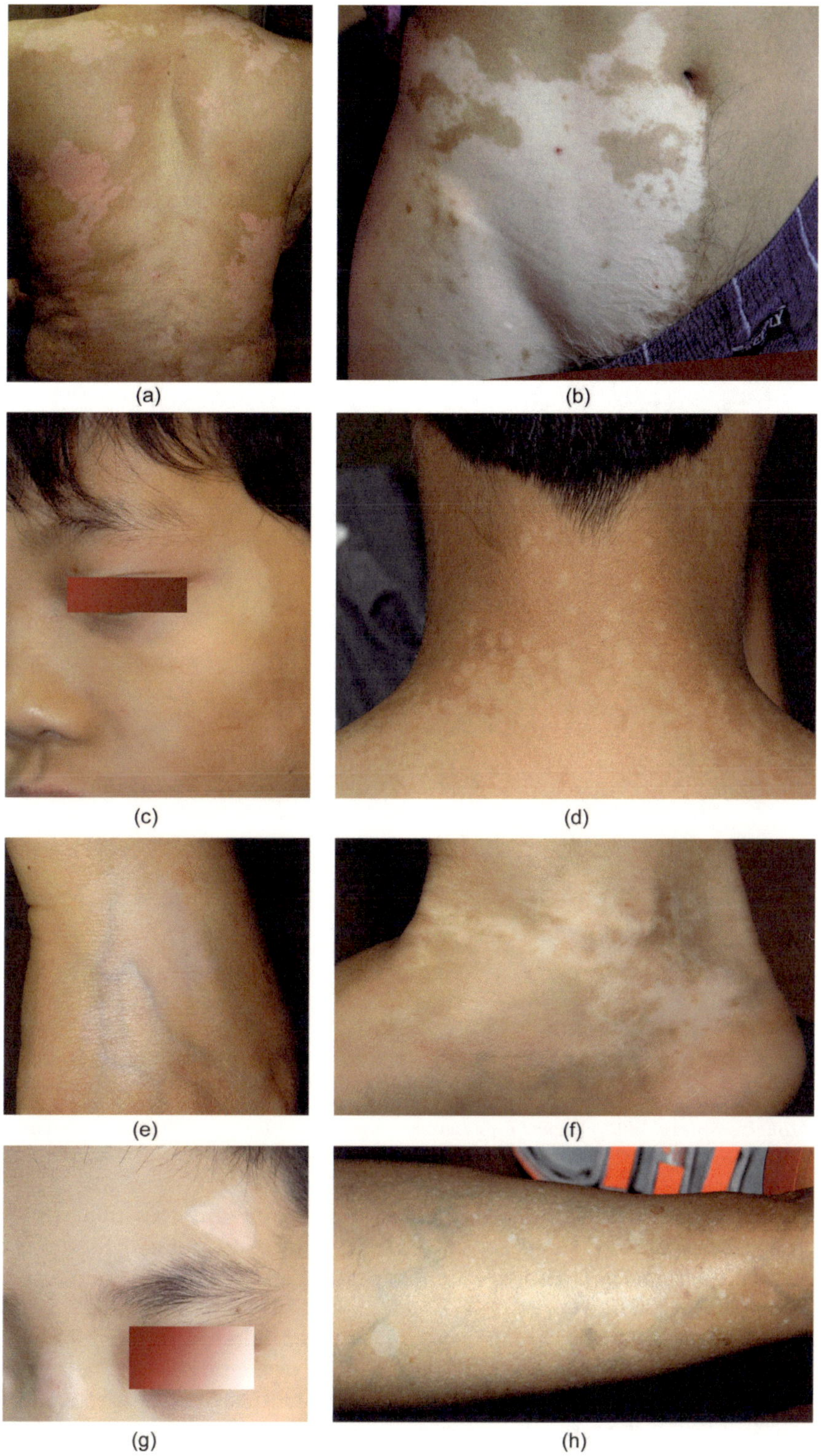

Figure 2.
Acquired diseases of depigmentation. a. Systemic vitiligo affecting the whole body. b. Segmental vitiligo affecting one side of the body with white hairs (poliosis). c. Pityriasis alba, hypomelanosis secondary to cutaneous inflammation of atopic dermatitis. d. Hypomelanosis by tinea versicolor. e. Hypomelanosis by strong steroid (injection of triamcinolone acetonide). f. Hypomelanosis from physical injury induced by burn. g. Hypomelanosis from physical injury induced by abrasion wound. h. Idiopathic guttate hypomelanosis in older patients which belong to miscellaneous hypopigmentation.

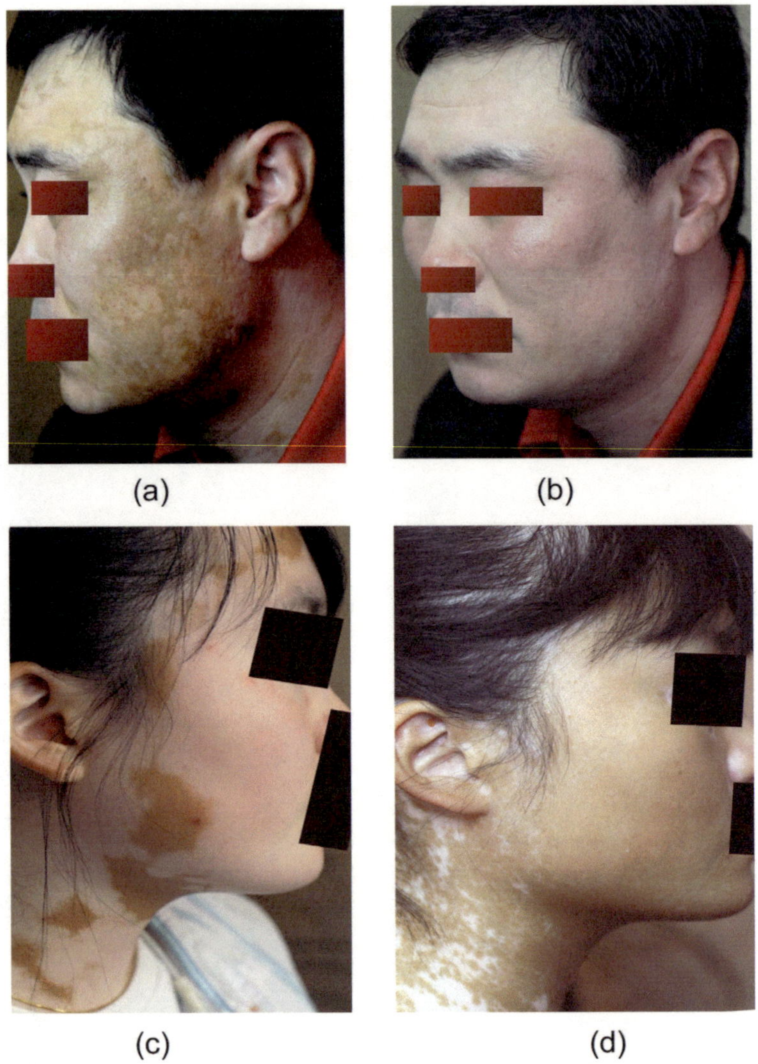

Figure 3.
Depigmentation therapies for vitiligo. a. Systemic vitiligo patient before depigmentation therapy by 20% monobenzyl-ether of hydroquinone (MBEH). b. Systemic vitiligo patient after 6 months of depigmentation therapy by 20% MBEH. c. Systemic vitiligo patient before 308 nm excimer laser therapy. d. Systemic vitiligo patient after 6 months of 308 nm excimer laser therapy.

As in **Figure 3a** and **b**, depigmentation therapy can be an ideal treatment for advanced vitiligo patients. But cases presented in **Figure 3c** and **d** suggests restoring normal pigmentation is also an excellent option, and it would be better to be decided by patient's choice.

Cosmeceutical for depigmentation is a big market field for investigators and cosmetic companies. We have tragedic experiencies of chemical leukoderma and vitiligo induced by depegmentation cometics manufactured by Kanebo containing rhododendrol [6, 7]. Researchers put tremendous efforts to overcome it and there are a lot of active researches to find out newer materials for depigmentation [4, 7].

DOI: http://dx.doi.org/10.5772/intechopen.89099

Author details

Tae-Heung Kim
White-Line Skin Clinic and Research Center, Changwon, Kyungnam, Korea

*Address all correspondence to: derkim@paran.com

References

[1] Wikipedia. Depigmentation. 2019. Available from: https://en.wikipedia.org/wiki/Depigmentation

[2] Choi S, Kim DY, Whang SH, Lee JH, Hann SK, Shin YJ. Quality of life and psychological adaptation of Korean adolescents with vitiligo. Journal of the European Academy of Dermatology and Venereology. 2010;**24**(5):524-529

[3] Passeron T, Ortonne J-P. Vitiligo and other disorders of hypopigmentation. In: Bolognia JL, Schaffer JV, Cerroni L, editors. Dermatology. 4th ed. Amsterdam, Netherlands: Elsevier Co; 2018. pp. 1087-1114

[4] Couteau C, Coiffard L. Overview of skin whitening agents: Drugs and cosmetic products. Cosmetics. 2016;**3**(3):27. https://doi.org/10.3390/cosmetics3030027

[5] Rodrigues M, Ezzedine K, Hamzavi I, Pandya AG, Harris JE, Vitiligo Working Group. Current and emerging treatments for vitiligo. Journal of the American Academy of Dermatology. 2017 Jul;**77**(1):17-29

[6] Harris JE. Chemical-induced vitiligo. Dermatologic Clinics. 2017;**35**(2):151-161

[7] Tokura Y, Fujiyama T, Ikeya S, Tatsuno K, Aoshima M, Kasuya A, et al. Biochemical, cytological, and immunological mechanisms of rhododendrol-induced leukoderma. Journal of Dermatological Science. 2015 Mar;**77**(3):146-149

Chapter 2

Lasers in the Treatment of Vitiligo

Isil Kamberoglu Turan

Abstract

Vitiligo is an acquired cutaneous hypopigmentary disorder characterized by multiple depigmented macules and patches. There are numerous therapy modalities consist of topical corticosteroids and calcineurin inhibitors, phototherapy, surgical interventions and laser treatments are evaluated. Last 10 years, firstly excimer laser treatment has showed good results in repigmentation rates. "Excited dimers" produces a 308-nm ultraviolet (UV) monochromatic coherent wavelength, which lies within the UVB spectrum that absorb DNA as a chromophore to breakage DNA chain that causes a decrease in T-lymphocyte proliferation. Some articles have shown different responses depends on the type of vitiligo, number of sessions, interval periods and localisation. Researchers have also compared efficacy and also side effects of excimer laser between other methods. Combination therapies with excimer laser will be also treatment of choice via topical steroids or topical calcineurin inhibitors. Some of the patients developed delayed-onset permanent hypopigmentation need resurfacing methods such as CO_2 or Er:YAG laser which mainly aims to ablate the epidermis in specific coagulation columns to promote the penetration of externally applied agent. As an alternative treatment modality in vitiligo, lasers may help to raise patient compliance and reduce potential risk for skin cancer. Its convenience is limited by high cost and accessibility.

Keywords: vitiligo, treatment, excimer, laser, refractory, CO_2

1. Introduction

Vitiligo is an autoimmune skin disorder with a 0.5–2.0% incidence worldwide without sex or age. It is characterized by hypopigmented macules and patches due to dysfunction of melanocytes. Etiology of the disease could not elucidated yet. The significant association between vitiligo and other autoimmune diseases, including alopecia areata, diabetes mellitus, Addison's disease, pernicious anemia, Graves' disease, Hashimoto's thyroiditis, systemic lupus erythematosus, rheumatoid arthritis, psoriasis and inflammatory bowel disease. Vitiliginous patches are often psychologically distressing and also have risk to loss of social status so that they cause negative impact of quality of life index. Two major forms are generally recognized that are *segmental* and *nonsegmental* types. Treatment of vitiligo is challenging and consensus of treatment modalities have changed beyond the types and places where the lesions mainstay. There are various phototherapy treatments which consist of PUVA, narrow-band UVB (NUVB), excimer laser and lamp commonly based on stimulation of melanocytes in the outer root sheath of hair follicles and on the margins of lesions besides that residual intralesional melanocytes migrate and repopulate the vitiliginous areas. Topical corticosteroid, calcineurin inhibitors, vitamine E and pseudocatalase could combine with these modalities to increase treatment response. Furthermore in stable vitiligo patients, surgical methods such as full-thickness tissue graft (punch graft), split thickness graft, and suction blister graft, cellular grafts contains cultured melanocytes/keratinocytes have shown promising results [1, 2].

2. Laser treatments approach in vitiligo patients

2.1 Excimer laser for immunomodulation in adult vitiligo patients

Monochromatic excimer light was first described for the treatment of psoriasis in 1997 and 4 years later Baltás et al. reported the first case of successful use of the excimer laser for the treatment of vitiligo in 2001 [3]. In vitiligo patients, the widely use narrowband UVB (NUVB) that contains 310–313 nm wavelength has safety profile. At that wavelength arrival we can also conduct monochromatic excimer laser (MEL) with an obligation of limited skin areas to protect nonlesional apart. Mostly clinicians uses 308 nm wavelength according to obtain skin epidermal barrier to induce immunotargeted therapy. New concept of era called targeted phototherapy is usually recommended for localized forms of vitiligo affecting less than 10% of the body surface area. Although these localized modality could prevent hyperpigmentation of uninvolved skin, it could not achieve to deprive new lesion output. In the literature we do not have so much scientific verifications. In Egypt, Eldin et al. *analyzed* 30 patients with nonsegmental vitiligo with at least two symmetrical vitiliginous patches. They treated twice a week for 6 weeks with 308-nm MEL and NUVB for 6 weeks these contralateral lesions. Three punch biopsies were taken from baseline and 6 weeks later. At the MEL group statistically significant rise in the number of basal pigmented cells in the earlier period [4]. According to that, MEL would be treatment of choice rather than NUVB because of rapid onset, lower cumulative doses and lesser treatment sessions. This study is the only proof of histopathological verification for comparison of these proven treatment modalities. Narrowband UVB, excimer laser and lamp has spreaded out similar wavelength even though they have different radiation properties. Mostly articles have shown that excimer laser and lamp have similar repigmentation rate and also minimal side effects so that clinicians should decide how to treat due to cost benefit analysis.

Lopes et al. published a metanalysis, they conducted there is no difference between repigmentation rate for all three treatment options. 308 nm excimer laser has much more safety profile than narrowband UVB because it works lesser time without affecting uninvolved skin and also affect deeper skin via changeable impulse frequency and intensity. However, excimer laser is characterized by monochromatic, coherent, and high-energy light, whereas NB-UVB consists of polychromatic, incoherent light with lower intensity [5]. Yan et al. declared that lesions located on the face and neck had better repigmentation rate with excimer lamp controversially extremities have better response with NB-UVB. Le Duff et al. observed that the excimer lamp is less expensive than the laser, allowing cost/effectiveness prolificacy however treatment period has been longer [6]. Sun et al. presented a scientifically supportive study such as seven randomized controlled trials. They declined that excimer laser has as similar as therapeutic effects with lamp and also combination of 308-nm excimer laser with 0.1% tacrolimus or with tacalcitol ointment can improve the repigmentation rate [7]. Different responses could be based on different angle of UVB-light emission to epidermis via fiber optic devices of excimer laser. Mostly, narrowband UVB treatment is used the most effective for nonsegmental vitiligo, while excimer laser treatment is commonly chosen for localized vitiligo by clinicians.

Efficacy of the excimer laser depends the number of session in a week or total cumulative doses. Fitzpatrick skin types of III and above typically respond better than lower skin types. As usual, facial, neck and axillary regions have quick response opposed to acral parts of body. Clinicians should refer minimal erythema dose (MED) and increment arrival differs between 10 and 25%. Frequency of the laser did not play a role in pigmentation although rapid onset of treatment depends on suitable action plan. Shen et al. determined that time of repigmentation begins earlier as same as in 2.0 and 3.0 frequency period than 1.0 but also all of them have same pigmentation areas [8]. According to small spot size, these modality is not suitable for patients with vitiligo involving large body surface areas (>15%). Repigmentation differs site by site consist of perifollicular, diffuse, marginal, and combined. The perifollicular pattern was the most common seen.

There is a negative correlation between the duration of the disease and the percentage of repigmentation which could be named as unresponsiveness. Topical corticosteroids have been a mainstay in vitiligo treatment for decades. However refractory vitiligo patients should need combination modalities. As known, topical corticosteroids have significant adverse effects such as skin atrophy, striae, erythema, acne, increased glucose level, glaucoma. According to that, topical pimecrolimus or tacrolimus ointments have been promising for the treatment of choice. Shin et al. would like to analyze combination of NUVB and excimer laser to unresponsive patients, they also determined that acral lesions are difficult part to treat but combination could be greater choice due to less adverse effect to difficult cases mainly in facial vitiligo group [9]. Latif et al. investigated two randomly selected vitiliginous patches, first group of lesions had taken combination of excimer laser and betamethasone dipropionate and calcipotriol ointment twice daily and second group had taken only excimer laser two unconsecutive days in a week for 12 weeks. They concluded that in nonsegmental vitiligo lesions treated with topical combination of vitamin D3 analogue and steroid with 308 nm MEL gave significant results rather than excimer laser alone and it could be promising option for the treatment of vitiligo [10]. All 10 patients who have bilateral symmetric vitiliginous patches received xenon chloride excimer laser three times weekly and calcipotriol ointment was applied twice Daily one side of the body. While conversely, during the 15th month follow up Goldinger et al. compared a combination of excimer laser and calcipotriol with excimer laser alone, and found no significant difference between them [11]. Passeron et al. analyzed the efficacy of combined tacrolimus (twice daily) and 380 nm excimer laser (twice a week) or difference of monotherapy. Twenty three lesions had taken excimer laser and tacrolimus combination but also 20 lesions had taken laser monotherapy and all lesions have similar repigmentation rates such as 100 versus 85%. They determined that UV-sensitive areas do not have different response rate but in UV-resistant areas combination treatment is clearly superior to laser monotherapy via synergistic effects [12]. Park et al. have shown that increment at the molecular level of tyrosinase and melanin in human melanocytes with combination of excimer laser and tacrolimus rather than each monotherapy in the first 6 month. However, this superiority was not observed in the patients who treated more than 6 months [13]. Wang et al. published an article, all patients received laser therapy twice weekly combined with tacrolimus cream twice daily for 12 weeks. Dermoscopy is a useful tool for asses the outcome of the laser. They found statistically significant induction of residual perifollicular pigmentation and perilesional hyperpigmentation in active disease rather than stable disease [14]. Topical antioxidant cream which includes superoxide dismutase and catalase activity could combine with excimer laser. Soliman et al. published an article the comparison of excimer laser alone and antioxidant cream combination via 30 patients have similar vitiliginous patches has followed up maximum 24 sessions, they found excellent cosmetic results regard minimal side effects [15] Bapur et al.

also has propagated topical tacrolimus or topical clobetasol-17 propionate ointment enhance the efficacy of excimer laser [16]. As a summary, there is big gap for to discuss which topical choice has better results.

In segmental vitiligo patients, excimer laser has claimed as a treatment of choice. As a proof, Bae et al. made a treatment schedule that received 20 mg of prednisolone daily for the first 3 weeks, twice a week excimer laser and twice a day tacrolimus ointment. They found more than half of the patients with segmental vitiligo showed 75% or more repigmentation with combination therapy for mean period is 1 year [17]. Jag et al. also investigate small sample size, firstly gave low-dose oral prednisolone (0.3 mg/kg/day) for 4–8 weeks, 0.1% topical tacrolimus twice daily, and excimer laser twice a week for 12 weeks. They found higher response rate rather than current therapies [18].

Bae et al. evaluated 311 Titanium-Sapphire Laser (TSL) Treatment in vitiligo that based on 14 patients with non-segmental vitiligo are treated with TSL twice a week. They determined working principle as similar as NUVB an EL by immunomodulation and melanocyte stimulation. Main advantage is not necessary to check gas charging and also penetrate deeper than 308 nm wavelength of excimer laser [19].

BinSheikan et al. suggested a surgical needling technique means 30 Gauge inserted almost parallel to the skin surface towards the dermoepidermal junction moving towards the pigmented site to depigmented skin could increase the efficacy of excimer laser [20]. Mutairi et al. reported that combination of split-skin grafting from normal skin to vitiligo part with excimer laser twice a week have long-lasting good results in stable vitiligo patients. All of them satisfied to treatment and respond excellent as well [21].

Leukotrichia also called poliosis mainstays white hair involving the scalp, eyebrows, and pubis has frequently seen together with segmental vitiligo. Kim et al. evaluated the effect of the presence of leukotrichia on the response to excimer laser therapy at the first time and they suggested that leukotrichia has poor response due to lack of melanocyte reservoir. They also did not find any difference between vitiligo types [22]. All in all, disease duration longer than 12 months, presence of leukotrichia and plurisegmental subtype were identified to be independent poor prognostic factors for excimer laser treatment.

Adverse effects of treatments are mild and acceptable which are pruritus, burning sensation, and dryness. MEL has a favorable risk-to-benefit ratio which has only minimal side effects are mainly acute and self-limited phototoxicity especially erythema does not persist longer than 24 hours. Furthermore another local site effects are tolerable that consist of blisters, itching or perilesional pigmentation but do not seen frequently.

If the patient does not improve meanly after 30 sessions twice or three times weekly, it is suggested that further treatment could provide any significant response [23].

Dermatology quality of life index (DLQI) scale could provide us convenient and important data for benefits of the treatment. It occasionally contained validated questionnaires such as symptoms and feelings, daily activities, leisure, work and school, personal relationships and treatment. In some analysis reports has concluded that long duration of disease, hand and face lesions and female patient have greater impairment of life index but also Shobaili et al. has shown that excimer laser has better improvement in quality of life index [25]. Alghamdi et al. made a survey in Saudi Arabia to prove dermatologists' clinical assessment for vitiligo treatment. They found excimer laser was the most common modality used to treat focal and segmental vitiligo and occasionally used in private clinics [26].

Excimer laser treatments respond faster recovery period and induce repigmentation rate so that clinicians use fewer treatments with less cumulative dose in order to achieve repigmentation compared with traditional phototherapy. The best result is noticed on UV-sensitive areas and also does not affect unlesional part of the body regard as the face and neck; whose has shorter history of vitiligo. Combination with topical steroid or topical calcineurin inhibitor (tacrolimus and pimecrolimus) increases the efficacy. The excimer laser has proven to be a useful tool in the treatment of vitiligo.

2.2 Excimer laser in child vitiligo patients

NBUVB is a safe and effective, well-tolerated treatment option for childhood vitiligo as well as for vitiligo in adults declared as a treatment of choice. Besides the adult population, children who has vitiligo also treated with excimer laser that based on xenon chloride lasers has been delivering radiation of 308–310 nm, with a variable spot size. Acral regions, resistant areas, hidden places are favorable for excimer laser. Gianfaldoni et al. determined treatment schedule should consist of twice weekly among 13 weeks to achieve good response [27]. Clinicians should estimate minimal erythema dose (MED) and begin with 10% lesser than it. Occasionally, face and neck has responded well but acral lesions has repigmented slowly. Cho et al. suggested that treatment response rate has correlated with anatomic site of the vitiligo lesion especially in localized type [28].

2.3 UVA1 target laser in children

Another optional treatment modality could regard as UVA1 target laser consists of an active medium and a Neodymium-doped yttrium orthovanadate (Nd:YVO4) crystal that is “energetically pumped” by another laser with 808 nm wavelength divided sequentially second (532 nm) and third (355 nm) harmonic wavelength delivery. Laser Alba allows the treatment of limited boarded lesional skin areas so that clinician can use a more appropriate dose of energy, leading to shorter duration and less frequent treatment sessions. The treatment with Laser Alba 355 is well—tolerated and already known acute side effects, such as erythema or pruritus have rarely been described.

Furthermore, innovative modalities consist of excimer laser, focused microphototherapy and also Laser ALBA should investigate to create new options [27, 29].

2.4 Fractional CO_2 laser for ablation modalities

As you know, vitiligo therapy is challenging though there is no definitive cure regime. Ablation therapy has recently been coalesced into combination therapy for vitiligo. These ablation modalities contains dermabrasion, erbium-YAG resurfacing, and ablative CO_2 laser treatment. Ablation modalities are not curative but they are useful to induce Koebner phenomenon to increase curative topical regimes. Fractional ablative laser has worked as a principle of photothermolysis to moderate skin resurfacing. Firstly, beneficial effect of fractional CO_2 laser on vitiligo is postulated to detachment of epidermis will release of cytokines and growth factors for immune response that plays a role as mitogens for melanogenesis. Additionally, fractional CO_2 laser via photothermolysis could decrease to skin surface so that absorb topical treatments and also increase efficacy of narrowband UVB treatment. Koebner’s phenomenon defined as the development of isomorphic lesions at traumatized uninvolved skin due to that fractional modalities to be concluded follicular hyperpigmentation as a different addition for pathogenesis. King et al. published a metanalysis, they determined ablation modalities (ER-YAG or fractional CO_2 laser) manage faster and effective repigmentation than the traditional methods that have explained via four different such as more penetration, skin remodeling, melanocyte migration and cytokine secretion [30]. Despite of that Koebner phenomenon has not seen in stable lesions so that individual remedy should be chosen. In a recent article Yuan et al. aim to investigate three different fractional laser types. Ablative fractional laser consist of CO_2 lasers have much more satisfied results than non-ablative lasers [31]. On the contrary, Mofty et al. evaluated that TCA peeling depends on Koebner phenomenon redounded repigmentation is much more cheap, easier and effective than ablative CO_2 laser [32]. Lu Li et al. has tried different model with CO_2 laser. They applied sequentially CO_2 laser during half month interval and used twice daily betamethasone then took NUVB. They checked the response rate at the baseline, 3th and 6th month and also found repigmentation more than half of the patients to compare without betamethasone ointment. They suggested patient got tolerable pain and gain more satisfied repigmentation rate than ER YAG laser is expected [33]. Helou et al. concerned a different modality contains CO_2 laser three times 1 month apart following that sunlight tanning at least 2 hours has also significant results. These different opinions will be future play as an easy to apply due to cost-benefit analysis [34]. Nevertheless, there is no defined protocol for ablation to stimulate melanocyte transmission.

More advanced ablation modalities could combine with other topical remedies to optimize results. Feily et al. comprised two group stable refractory vitiligo patients got autologous transplantation and phototherapy alone or with fractional CO_2 laser. They found perifollicular repigmentation was statistically significant detectable in CO_2 laser group before the transplantation [35]. Vachiremon et al. suggested that fractional ablative CO_2 laser could combine with NUVB to shorten duration time of recovery and increase the penetration of light immunomodulation and also topical clobetasol propionate ointment [36]. Additionally that, acral part could not reach the treatments so that alternatives should try. By using CO_2 laser, clinicians have seen lesser hypertrophic scars than ERYAG laser also so that treatment of choice in ablative lasers could manifested. Mohamed et al. searched the combination of 5-Fluorouracil cream and CO_2 laser due to ablation of dermis to penetrate cream to migrate melanocytes in acral vitiligo patients. They declined that combination treatment is safe and tolerable technique for these resistant types [37]. Chen et al. investigated the topical tacrolimus combination with CO_2 laser, they suggested tacrolimus would be good option with ablation therapies, also [38]. Using with CO_2 laser, hypertrophic scarring was not reported because of the superficial ablation that means removing only the epidermis, avoiding the dermis.

As a summary, ablation-based combination therapy is safe and might be more effective than treatments without ablation therapy for increment of repigmentation.

2.5 Erbium laser for ablation modalities

The Er:YAG laser emits light at 2940 nm, with the water affinity being nearly 15 times greater than that of the CO_2 laser. Use of the Er:YAG laser requires more skill than does use of the CO_2 laser as the clinical endpoints allowing the laser surgeon require to intervene further penetration into the reticular dermis, are not seen with Er:YAG laser ablation. Furthermore, the plateau response of diminishing ablation characteristic of the CO_2 laser is not seen with the Er:YAG laser [1, 24]. Lotti et al. used a different innovation in a ablative model with Fraxel Erbium Laser (fractional erbium laser) make epidermal erosion 1 day after apply topical latanoprost solution and finally use UVA laser. The patients have nine sessions so on 90% of them obtained a repigmentation rate higher than 75% [39]. Bayoumi et al. tried to use erbium laser firstly for aiming dermabrasion after that 48 hours hydrocortisone 17-butyrate cream applied three times a day daily for 3 weeks followed by a 1-week steroid-free interval and narrowband UVB treatment was performed on both sides twice weekly for 12 weeks. They succeed in refractory lesions due to Koebner' phenomenon almost half of the lesions treated at least 50% repigmentation rate and more than 16% achieved a complete or almost complete repigmentation [40]. As a point of view, that difference from non-treated part, dermabrasion has induced penetration of UVB and topical steroid so it cause enhancement of melanocyte stimulation. For example Yan et al. have a different perspective they insisted on energy should be set at the level of at least 1200 mJ. They divided four parts such as one of them is control group given NUVB and other three of them took different frequency of energy to calibrate most effective and least painful method of these modality. They found better response at the medium or high energy protocols [41]. Mohtari et al. tried to find a unresponsiveness vitiligo part a new modality that is firstly used ER:YAG laser than applied clobetasol or 5-FU dressing and found better cosmetic results via ablation [42]. As expected, periungual vitiligo hard places to treat responded well. Two-thirds of the patients (66.7%) showed moderate to marked repigmentation via ER:YAG after dressing 5-FU [43].

On the whole, the acral regions were considered the most resistant to traditional treatment modalities. According to that, ER:YAG laser with topical corticoid, tacrolimus or 5-FU application could be promising treatment modality for unresponsiveness patients.

2.6 Q-switch laser for depigmentation modalities

Depigmentation is the unique treatment choice who develop vitiligo more than 90% body surface area, for the term "universal vitiligo" is commonly used. Topical agent such as MBEH (monobenzyl ether of hydroquinone) has main role to epidermal ablation and resurfacing. Laser therapies depend on therapies via difference to intact areas such as epidermal and dermal types. Specifically, Q switch laser could achieve faster depigmentation compared with chemical agents and the decrease the risk of scar formation. Q-switched Nd:YAG (QS ND:Yag) laser can deliver energy at two different wavelengths of 1064 and 532 nm in nanosecond pulses to cause both a photothermolytic and photoacoustic damage to melanocytes [1, 24].

Majid et al. followed up 15 patients covered more than 80% depigmentation areas whole body who have not respond MBEH least 3 months, They focused on Q-switch laser at 532 nm for epidermal component for need any session took 6th week arrival while continuing MBEH topical agents use has rapid onset improvement and minimal adverse effect [44]. Komen et al. has published a questionnaire about the result of Q switch (QS) Ruby laser that concluded 48% of the treated patients showed >75% depigmentation after a mean of 13 months' follow-up. This is the first study that comparison between active vitiligo during QS Ruby laser treatment have properly better results than stable vitiligo [45]. As a choice of MBEH, sometimes, the depigmentation site has gave up to fight immune system and looked more darker so that clinicians has to improve concentration. Modi et al. rather to use 532-nm Q-switched neodymium-doped yttrium aluminum garnet (QS Nd:Yag) laser via 2 sessions with 15 weeks intervals have good results. They offer to give 3 or 4 months apart to allow for maximal treatment response [46]. Majid et al. has followed up 25 patients with universal vitiligo from 2 to 5 years and determined QS-Nd:Yag laser leads to a long-term therapeutic effect in a majority of cases when used at 532-nm wavelength. Less than one third of cases during the follow-up period could preserve the therapeutic benefit achieved with laser treatment [47]. Boukari et al. has followed patients for 36 months depigmented 20 lesions via Q Switch laser and determined that risk of depigmentation parts mainstays in sun exposed areas have need maintenance therapies [48].

In conclusion, QS Nd:YAG laser at 532-nm wavelength seems to be a safe and effective treatment in depigmenting approach to universal vitiligo. The safety and long-term benefit achieved should qualify QS laser treatment as first-line treatment who did not respond topical bleaching creams. Moreover, QS laser combine with topical bleaching creams and sunscreen use, can achieve rapid satisfactory therapeutic outcome in universal vitiligo.

3. Conclusion

Vitiligo is a difficult disease to treat because of that new modalities should be investigated. As you known, traditional remedies such as NUVB and topical corticosteroids or tacrolimus did not respond well than new era has developed a concept called targeted phototherapy. Regarded as a targeted phototherapy excimer laser has same wavelength as same as NUVB to focused on apoptosis of T lymphocytes. However, excimer laser is characterized by monochromatic, coherent, and high-energy light, whereas NB-UVB consists of polychromatic, incoherent light with lower intensity. Excimer laser has significant safety profile and got better results than NUVB so that clinicians should decide the option to evaluate cost benefit analysis. Other traditional topical remedies could also apply with excimer laser to induce effectiveness. In segmental vitiligo patients or child population, excimer laser could be treatment of choice also due to localized areas. Another point of view of the laser treatment is ablation. Using the Koebner phenomenon, CO_2 laser and ER:YAG have worked as a principle of photothermolysis to moderate skin resurfacing. Traditional remedies could also combine with ablative laser types to increase the absorption of the treatments. Clinicians further to analyze depigmentation need. If patient has more than 80% depigmented areas, Q switch laser combine with topical bleaching creams and sunscreen use, can achieve rapid satisfactory therapeutic outcome in universal vitiligo. Vitiligo does not have a steady all known treatment protocols even though clinicians should further to investigate new combinations.

Author details

Isil Kamberoglu Turan
Dokuz Eylul University, Izmir, Turkey

*Address all correspondence to: isil.kamberoglu@gmail.com

References

[1] Bolognia JL, Joseph JL, Schaffer JV, editors. Dermatology. 4th ed. Philadelphia: Elsevier Saunders; 2018

[2] Al-Otaibi SR, Zadeh VB, Al-Abdulrazzaq AH, Tarrab SM, Al-Owaidi HA, Mahrous R, et al. Using a 308-nm excimer laser to treat vitiligo in Asians. Acta Dermatovenerologica Alpina, Pannonica et Adriatica. 2009;**18**(1):13-19

[3] Baltás E, Csoma Z, Ignácz F, Dobozy A, Kemény L. Treatment of vitiligo with the 308-nm xenon chloride excimer laser. Archives of Dermatology. 2002;**138**(12):1619-1620. DOI: 10.1001/archderm.138.12.1613

[4] Salah Eldin MM, Sami NA, Aly DG, Hanafy NS. Comparison between (311-312 nm) narrow band ultraviolet-B phototherapy and (308 nm) monochromatic excimer light phototherapy in treatment of Vitiligo: A histopathological study. Journal of Lasers in Medical Sciences. 2017;**8**(3):123-127. DOI: 10.15171/jlms.2017.22

[5] Lopes C, Trevisani VF, Melnik T. Efficacy and safety of 308-nm monochromatic excimer lamp versus other phototherapy devices for Vitiligo: A systematic review with meta-analysis. American Journal of Clinical Dermatology. 2016;**17**(1):23-32. DOI: 10.1007/s40257-015-0164-2

[6] Le Duff F, Fontas E, Giacchero D, Sillard L, Lacour JP, Ortonne JP, et al. 308-nm excimer lamp vs. 308-nm excimer laser for treating vitiligo: A randomized study. The British Journal of Dermatology. 2010;**163**(1):188-192. DOI: 10.1111/j.1365-2133.2010.09778.x

[7] Sun Y, Wu Y, Xiao B, Lu L, Li L, Chen H-D, et al. Treatment of 308 nm excimer laser on Vitiligo: A systemic review of randomized controlled trials. The Journal of Dermatological Treatment. 2015;**26**(4):347-353. DOI: 10.3109/09546634.2014.991268

[8] Shen Z, Gao TW, Chen L, Yang L, Wang YC, Sun LC, et al. Optimal frequency of treatment with the 308-nm excimer laser for vitiligo on the face and neck. Photomedicine and Laser Surgery. 2007;**25**(5):418-427

[9] Shin S, Hann SK, Oh SH. Combination treatment with excimer laser and narrowband UVB light in vitiligo patients. Photodermatology, Photoimmunology & Photomedicine. 2016;**32**(1):28-33. DOI: 10.1111/phpp.12212

[10] Abdel Latif AA, Ibrahim SM. Monochromatic excimer light versus combination of topical steroid with vitamin D3 analogue in the treatment of nonsegmental vitiligo: A randomized blinded comparative study. Dermatologic Therapy. 2015;**28**(6):383-389. DOI: 10.1111/dth.12289

[11] Goldinger SM, Dummer R, Schmid P, Burg G, Seifert B, Läuchli S. Combination of 308-nm xenon chloride excimer laser and topical calcipotriol in vitiligo. Journal of the European Academy of Dermatology and Venereology. 2007;**21**(4):504-508. DOI: 10.1111/j.1468-3083.2006.02016.x

[12] Passeron T, Ostovari N, Zakaria W, Fontas E, Larrouy JC, Lacour JP, et al. Topical tacrolimus and the 308-nm excimer laser: A synergistic combination for the treatment of vitiligo. Archives of Dermatology. 2004;**140**(9):1065-1069. DOI: 10.1001/archderm.140.9.1065

[13] Park OJ, Park GH, Choi JR, Jung HJ, Oh ES, Choi JH, et al. A combination of excimer laser treatment and topical tacrolimus is more effective in treating vitiligo than either therapy alone for

the initial 6 months, but not thereafter. Clinical and Experimental Dermatology. 2016;**41**(3):236-241. DOI: 10.1111/ced.12742

[14] Wang LM, Lu WJ, Yuan JT, Zeng BB, Li D, Zhang F, et al. Utility of dermoscopy for evaluating the therapeutic efficacy of tacrolimus ointment plus 308-nm excimer laser combination therapy in localized vitiligo patients. Experimental and Therapeutic Medicine. 2018;**15**(4):3981-3988. DOI: 10.3892/etm.2018.5911

[15] Soliman M, Samy NA, Abo Eittah M, Hegazy M. Comparative study between excimer light and topical antioxidant versus excimer light alone for treatment of vitiligo. Journal of Cosmetic and Laser Therapy. 2016;**18**(1):7-11. DOI: 10.3109/14764172.2015.1052510

[16] Bapur Erduran F, Adışen E. Comparison of the efficacy of 308-nm excimer lamp monotherapy with topical tacrolimus or clobetasol 17-propionate combination therapies in localized vitiligo. Photodermatology, Photoimmunology & Photomedicine. 2016;**32**(5-6):247-253. DOI: 10.1111/phpp.12266

[17] Bae JM, Yoo HJ, Kim H, Lee JH, Kim GM. Combination therapy with 308-nm excimer laser, topical tacrolimus, and short-term systemic corticosteroids for segmental vitiligo: A retrospective study of 159 patients. Journal of the American Academy of Dermatology. 2015;**73**(1):76-82. DOI: 10.1016/j.jaad.2015.04.008

[18] Jang YH, Jung S-E, Shin J, Kang HY. Triple combination of systemic corticosteroids, excimer laser, and topical tacrolimus in the treatment of recently developed localized vitiligo. Annals of Dermatology. 2015;**27**(1):104-107. DOI: 10.5021/ad.2015.27.1.104

[19] Bae JM, Lee JH, Jung YS, Kim GM. The efficacy of gain-switched 311-nm titanium: Sapphire laser in the treatment of Vitiligo: A pilot study of 14 patients. JAMA Dermatology. 2017;**153**(10):1055-1056. DOI: 10.1001/jamadermatol.2017.2175

[20] BinSheikhan S, Al Abadie M. Improvement in moderate to severe vitiligo using a novel combination of 308 nm excimer laserand a surgical needling technique. Clinical and Experimental Dermatology. 2017;**42**(3):363-366. DOI: 10.1111/ced.13056

[21] Al-Mutairi N, Manchanda Y, Al-Doukhi A, Al-Haddad A. Long-term results of split-skin grafting in combination with excimer laser for stable vitiligo. Dermatologic Surgery. 2010;**36**(4):499-505. DOI: 10.1111/j.1524-4725.2010.01477.x

[22] Kim MS, Cho EB, Park EJ, Kim KH, Kim KJ. Effect of excimer laser treatment on vitiliginous areas with leukotrichia after confirmation by dermoscopy. International Journal of Dermatology. 2016;**55**(8):886-892. DOI: 10.1111/ijd.12972

[23] Hamzavi IH, Lim HW, Syed ZU. Ultraviolet based therapy for vitiligo: What's new? Indian Journal of Dermatology, Venereology and Leprology. 2012;**78**(1):42-48. DOI: 10.4103/0378-6323.90945

[24] Goldberg DJ. Laser Dermatology. 2th ed. DOI: 10.1007/978-3-642-32006-4

[25] Al-Shobaili HA. Treatment of vitiligo patients by excimer laser improves patients' quality of life. Journal of Cutaneous Medicine and Surgery. 2015;**19**(1):50-56. DOI: 10.2310/7750.2014.14002

[26] Al Ghamdi KM, Khurram H, Taïeb A. Survey of dermatologists' phototherapy practices for vitiligo. Indian Journal of Dermatology, Venereology and

Leprology. 2012;**78**:74-81. DOI: 10.4103/0378-6323.90950

[27] Gianfaldoni S, Tchernev G, Wollina U, Lotti J, Rovesti M, Satolli F, et al. Vitiligo in children: What's new in treatment? Open Access Macedonian Journal of Medical Sciences. 2018;**6**(1):221-225. DOI: 10.3889/oamjms.2018.060

[28] Cho S, Kang HC, Hahm JH. Characteristics of vitiligo in Korean children. Pediatric Dermatology. 2000;**17**(3):189-193

[29] Lotti T, Tchernev G, Wollina U, França K, Lotti J, Satolli F, et al. Successful treatment with UVA 1 laser of non-responder Vitiligo patients. Open Access Macedonian Journal of Medical Sciences. 2018;**6**(1):43-45. DOI: 10.3889/oamjms.2018.047

[30] King YA, Tsai TY, Tsai HH, Huang YC. The efficacy of ablation based combination therapy for vitiligo: A systematic review and meta-analysis. Journal der Deutschen Dermatologischen Gesellschaft. 2018;**16**(10):1197-1208. DOI: 10.1111/ddg.13657

[31] Yuan J, Chen H, Yan R, Cui S, Li YH, Wu Y, et al. Fractional CO_2 lasers contribute to the treatment of stable non-segmental vitiligo. European Journal of Dermatology. 2016;**26**(6):592-598. DOI: 10.1684/ejd.2016.2875

[32] El Mofty M, Esmat S, Hunter N, Mashaly HM, Dorgham D, Shaker O, et al. Effect of different types of therapeutic trauma on vitiligo lesions. Dermatologic Therapy. 2017;**30**(2). DOI: 10.1111/dth.12447

[33] Li L, Wu Y, Li L, Sun Y, Qiu L, Gao XH, et al. Triple combination treatment with fractional CO_2 laser plus topical betamethasone solution and narrowband ultraviolet B for refractory vitiligo: A prospective, randomized half-body, comparative study. Dermatologic Therapy. 2015;**28**(3): 131-134. DOI: 10.1111/dth.12202

[34] Hélou J, Maatouk I, Obeid G, Moutran R, Stéphan F, Tomb R. Fractional laser for vitiligo treated by 10,600 nm ablative fractional carbon dioxide laser followed by sun exposure. Lasers in Surgery and Medicine. 2014;**46**(6):443-448. DOI: 10.1002/lsm.22260

[35] Feily A, Seifi V, Ramirez-Fort MK. Fractional CO_2 laser pretreatment to autologous hair transplantation and phototherapy improves perifollicular repigmentation in refractory Vitiligo: A randomized, prospective, half-lesion, comparative study. Dermatologic Surgery. 2016;**42**(9):1082-1088. DOI: 10.1097/DSS.0000000000000844

[36] Vachiramon V, Chaiyabutr C, Rattanaumpawan P, Kanokrungsee S. Effects of a preceding fractional carbon dioxide laser on the outcome of combined local narrowband ultraviolet B and topical steroids in patients with vitiligo in difficult-to-treat areas. Lasers in Surgery and Medicine. 2016;**48**(2):197-202. DOI: 10.1002/lsm.22389

[37] Mohamed HA, Mohammed GF, Gomaa AH, Eyada MM. Carbon dioxide laser plus topical 5-fluorouracil: A new combination therapeutic modality for acral vitiligo. Journal of Cosmetic and Laser Therapy. 2015;**17**(4):216-223. DOI: 10.3109/14764172.2014.1003241

[38] Chen W, Zhou Y, Huang FR, Luo D, Wang DG. Preliminary study on the treatment of vitiligo with carbon dioxide fractional laser together with tacrolimus. Lasers in Surgery and Medicine. 2018;**50**(8):829-836. DOI: 10.1002/lsm.22821

[39] Lotti T, Wollina U, Tchernev G, Valle Y, Lotti J, França K, et al. An innovative therapeutic protocol for Vitiligo:

Experience with the use of Fraxel herbium laser, topical latanoprost and successive irradiation with UVA-1 laser. Open Access Macedonian Journal of Medical Sciences. 2018;**6**(1):49-51. DOI: 10.3889/oamjms.2018.059

[40] Bayoumi W, Fontas E, Sillard L, Le Duff F, Ortonne JP, Bahadoran P, et al. Effect of a preceding laser dermabrasion on the outcome of combined therapy with narrowband ultraviolet B and potent topical steroids for treating nonsegmental vitiligo in resistant localizations. The British Journal of Dermatology. 2012;**166**(1):208-211. DOI: 10.1111/j.1365-2133.2011.10564.x

[41] Yan R, Yuan J, Chen H, Li YH, Wu Y, Gao XH, et al. Fractional Er:YAG laser assisting topical betamethasone solution in combination with NB-UVB for resistant non-segmental vitiligo. Lasers in Medical Science. 2017;**32**(7):1571-1577. DOI: 10.1007/s10103-017-2282-y

[42] Mokhtari F, Bostakian A, Shahmoradi Z, Jafari-Koshki T, Iraji F, Faghihi G, et al. Potential emerging treatment in vitiligo using Er:YAG in combination with 5FU and clobetasol. Journal of Cosmetic Dermatology. 2018;**17**(2):165-170. DOI: 10.1111/jocd.12373

[43] Anbar T, Westerhof W, Abdel-Rahman A, El-Khayyat M, El-Metwally Y. Treatment of periungual vitiligo with erbium-YAG-laser plus 5-flurouracil: A left to right comparative study. Journal of Cosmetic Dermatology. 2006;**5**(2):135-139. DOI: 10.1111/j.1473-2165.2006.00240.x

[44] Majid I, Imran S. Depigmentation therapy with Q-switched Nd: YAG laser in universal Vitiligo. Journal of Cutaneous and Aesthetic Surgery. 2013;**6**(2):93-96. DOI: 10.4103/0974-2077.112670

[45] Komen L, Zwertbroek L, Burger SJ, van der Veen JP, de Rie MA, Wolkerstorfer A. Q-switched laser depigmentation in vitiligo, most effective in active disease. The British Journal of Dermatology. 2013;**169**(6):1246-1251. DOI: 10.1111/bjd.12571

[46] Modi K, Mohammad TF, Hamzavi IH. Use of the 532-nm Q-switched neodymium-doped yttrium aluminum garnet laser for the treatment of recalcitrant repigmentation in vitiligo. JAAD Case Reports. 2018;**4**(6):612-614. DOI: 10.1016/j.jdcr.2018.04.010

[47] Majid I, Imran S. Depigmentation with Q-switched Nd:YAG laser in universal vitiligo: A long-term follow-up study of 4 years. Lasers in Medical Science. 2017;**32**(4):851-855. DOI: 10.1007/s10103-017-2183-0

[48] Boukari F, Lacour JP, Ortonne JP, Bahadoran P, Passeron T. Laser-assisted depigmentation for resistant vitiligo: A retrospective case series with long-term follow-up. Journal of the European Academy of Dermatology and Venereology. 2014;**28**(3):374-377. DOI: 10.1111/jdv.12038

Chapter 3

Histopathology and Molecular Pathology of Vitiligo

Amit Kumar Yadav

Abstract

Vitiligo is a common skin disorder that manifests as whitish macules. There is no special geographic or sex predilection. Vitiligo is a multifactorial disorder. The various theories proposed include neutral theory, autoimmune theory, zinc-α2-glycoprotein theory, viral infection, intrinsic theory and melanocytorrhagy theory. However, the currently favored opinion is that there is a convergence of various theories known as the convergence theory. The basic defect is the absence of functional melanocytes from the epidermal melanin unit. This absence can be demonstrated by using special stains like Fontana-Masson, immunohistochemistry like HMB-45 and Melan-A and electron microscopy. Margins of lesions especially early lesions show inflammatory cells principally CD4+ and CD8+ T cells. The cornerstone of management in vitiligo is correct categorization of a case into stable and unstable vitiligo. This distinction is based mainly on clinical criteria. It is recommended that while evaluating biopsies, histopathological examination should be primarily concentrated on evaluating five histopathological variables—spongiosis, epidermal lymphocytes, basal cell vacuolation, dermal lymphocytes and melanophages. These parameters are then scored using a scoring system, and the recommended diagnoses based on these scores are given. Adoption of a systematic reporting system brings more consistency and objectivity in the diagnosis.

Keywords: vitiligo, multifactorial, convergence theory, melanocytes, histological scoring

1. Introduction

Vitiligo is a common acquired, idiopathic, progressive disorder which is characterized by the development of depigmented milky white macules of variable sizes. These often enlarge and coalesce to form extensive areas of leukoderma [1–3]. It equally affects both sexes with a worldwide prevalence of 0.1–2% [4]. It is a psychologically devastating and frequently resistant to treatment [5, 6]. The basic defect in vitiligo is a selective destruction of functional melanocytes [7].

The role of histopathology in the diagnosis of vitiligo is not yet fully established. So much so that routinely in these cases biopsy is not performed. The diagnosis is made primarily on clinical grounds.

 IntechOpen

2. Pathogenesis

Vitiligo is a multifactorial disorder [8, 9]. In its genesis both genetic and non-genetic factors are believed to play a role. It is observed that clinically no two patients of vitiligo are alike. This suggests that etiology also varies among different patients. Due to the observed variation in clinical manifestations of the disease, it seems likely that etiology of vitiligo may differ among patients [10]. These several theories have been combined into the convergence theory [11] which is currently the most accepted theory.

Briefly in the earliest theory, it was proposed by Lerner that vitiligo was neural in origin [12]. This theory could explain the segmental form of vitiligo which follows dermatomal distribution and is associated with hyperhidrosis and emotional disturbances. In another study the role of sympathetic nervous system in vitiligo was studied [13]. It was observed that the cutaneous blood flow in the lesional skin was three times higher than the normal skin in cases of segmental vitiligo. However, in other cases of non-segmental vitiligo, this was not observed.

Studies on the expression of neural proteins like neuropeptide Y (NPY), calcitonin gene-related peptide (CGRP), vasoactive intestinal polypeptide (VIP) and polyclonal general neuronal marker (PGP) have shown variable results. In one study NPY expression was found to be increased in cases of segmental vitiligo [14]. It is proposed that precipitating factors like stress lead to increased NPY expression [15].

But this theory failed to explain the other forms of vitiligo. For that matter generalized or non-segmental vitiligo is better explained by autoimmune hypothesis. In previously done studies, antibodies against various targets like tyrosine hydroxylase, melanin-concentrating hormone receptor-1 (MCHR1), tyrosinase [16] and pigment cell surface antigens [17] have been demonstrated. In a study carried out to evaluate the various immunoglobulins, it was observed that 80% of active vitiligo patients showed the presence of IgG and IgM against melanocytes [17]. Other studies have shown the presence of anti-thyroglobulin antibodies, antithyroid antibodies, anti-thyroperoxidase and anti-smooth muscle antibody in these cases [18, 19].

Besides humoral immunity, cell-mediated immunity may also play an important role. Immunohistochemical examination of perilesional skin in vitiligo patients showed increased CD8:CD4 ratio and HLA-DR production along suprabasal and basal keratinocytes. Macrophages were found to be quite numerous [20]. However, not only the immune cells and antibodies but expression of various cytokines is also increased. Chief among these which have been studied are tumor necrosis factor-α (TNF-α), interferon-γ (IFN-γ) and IL-10 [21, 22]. IL-17 has also been shown to be significantly increased in cases of vitiligo [23].

The redox (reduction–oxidation) state of vitiliginous patients has been studied by many authors. These studies have shown increased serum levels of selenium, superoxide dismutase (SOD) and malondialdehyde (MDA) [24, 25]. Increased levels of these substances indicate the presence of oxidative stress in vitiligo. Increased levels of tetrahydrobiopterin [26] and xanthine oxidase [27] leading to increased levels of H_2O_2 may also be contributory.

Few authors have pointed towards the role of zinc-α2-glycoprotein (ZAG) in the pathogenesis of vitiligo. They hypothesize that lack of ZAG causes impaired melanocytic adhesion to other cells in the epidermis [28, 29]. The efficacy of zinc in the treatment of vitiligo may be due to its ability to precipitate ZAG at the site of vitiligo [30].

The role of viral infection in vitiligo has been proposed by certain authors. The potential candidates include hepatitis C virus (HCV) [31], cytomegalovirus (CMV) [32], Epstein–Barr virus (EBV), hepatitis e virus, herpes virus and HIV [33]. However, the evidence available is scant and not conclusive enough to attribute a significant role for viral agents in vitiligo.

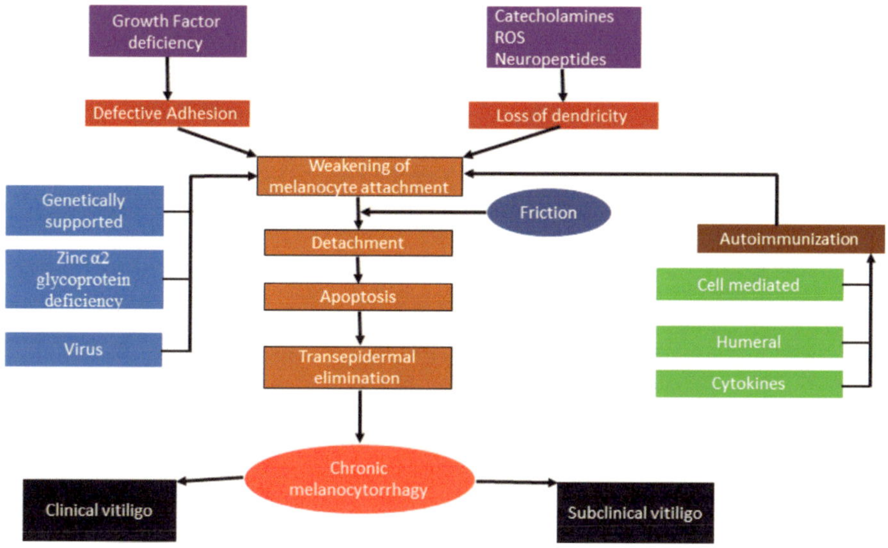

Figure 1.
Pathogenesis of vitiligo.

The intrinsic theory states that in vitiligo there is loss of melanocytes due to various abnormalities which lead to increased apoptosis [34] and accelerated cell senescence [35, 36]. Studies done previously have shown various abnormalities in the melanocytes including cytoplasmic vacuolization, DNA marginalization, dendrite loss and detachment [36, 37]. The evidence in favor of increased apoptosis in vitiligo includes reduced expression levels of the antiapoptotic proteins Bcl-2 and FLIP in vitiliginous skin as compared to normal skin [34]. On the other hand, marked increase in the expression of proapoptotic factors such as Bax and p53 along with the various caspases has also been observed [34].

The melanocytorrhagy theory states that in vitiligo there is chronic melanocyte detachment and loss caused by trauma and other stressors which include catecholamines, free radicals or autoimmune elements [38].

However, the consensus opinion of majority of experts is that vitiligo occurs due to convergence of these various pathways [39]. These are also depicted in (**Figure 1**). The author also is in agreement with this view; however, it is likely that in various subtypes of vitiligo the relative contribution of these pathways may vary. For example, in segmental vitiligo the neural theory may be more relevant than the other theories, whereas the same may not hold true for vitiligo vulgaris.

3. Histopathology

In order to understand the histopathology of vitiligo, it is essential to first understand the concept of *epidermal melanin unit* [40]. Melanocytes are neural crest derivatives, and they reach their final destination of basal layer of the epidermis and hair follicles via a process of migration. Each melanocyte then transfers its melanosomes to approximately 36 keratinocytes via a unique mechanism known as the shedding vesicle system. In the normal skin in the basal layer of the epidermis for every five basal keratinocytes, there is a presence of a single melanocyte [41].

The basic histopathological finding in vitiligo is the absence of functional melanocytes in the basal layer of the epidermis (**Figure 2**) [42–44]. This absence can also be demonstrated by using special stains like Fontana-Masson (**Figure 3**) [45].

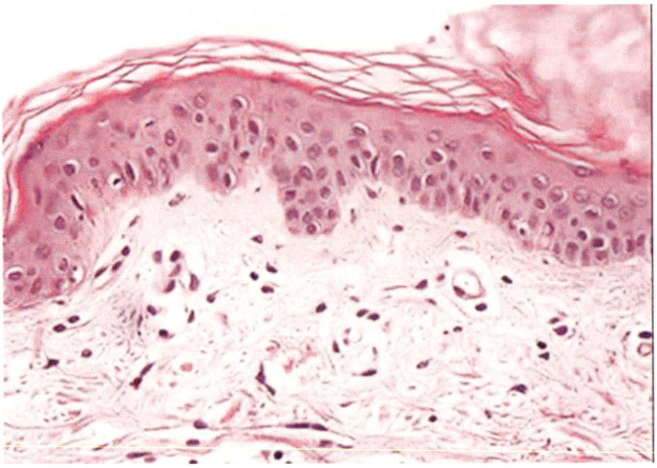

Figure 2.
Vitiligo showing the absence of melanocytes in basal layer of the epidermis (H&E, X400).

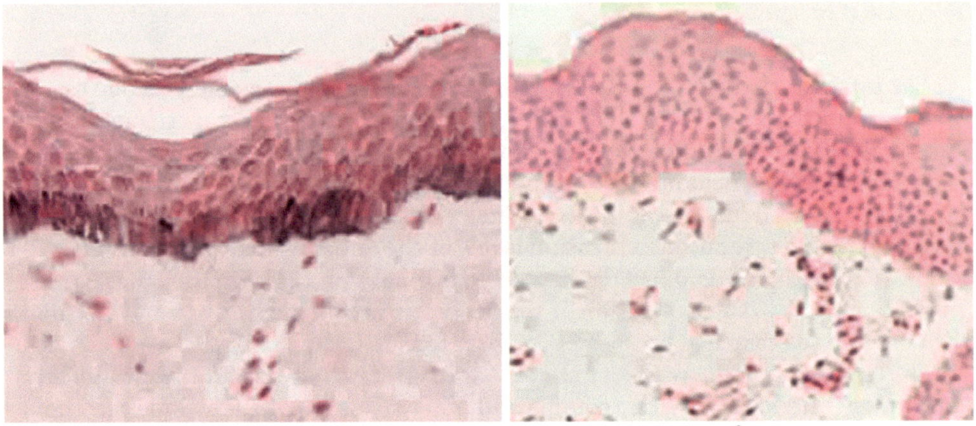

a b

Figure 3.
(a) Fontana-Masson showing the presence of melanin pigment and melanocytes in the epidermis (X400).
(b) Fontana-Masson showing the absence of melanin pigment and melanocytes in the epidermis (x400).

Immunohistochemistry for melanocyte-specific markers like HMB-45 and Melan-A and electron microscopy can also be performed for this purpose.

Other changes that have been observed include degenerative changes in the nerves and adnexa like sebaceous glands and hair follicles especially in long-standing cases [46].

In the margins of lesions especially early lesions, often inflammatory cells are seen. Principally, these cells comprise of CD4+ and CD8+ T cells [47]. These cells have been shown to demonstrate melanocyte-specific cytotoxicity [48]. At the margins of the lesions, melanocytes have been observed to show morphological changes like cellular enlargement, cytoplasmic vacuolization and long dendritic processes [29].

However, usually skin biopsy is not performed for making the diagnosis as it is primarily a clinical diagnosis. The cornerstone of its management is correct categorization of a case into its two broad types—stable and unstable vitiligo. This distinction is at present based mainly on clinical criteria because the histopathological

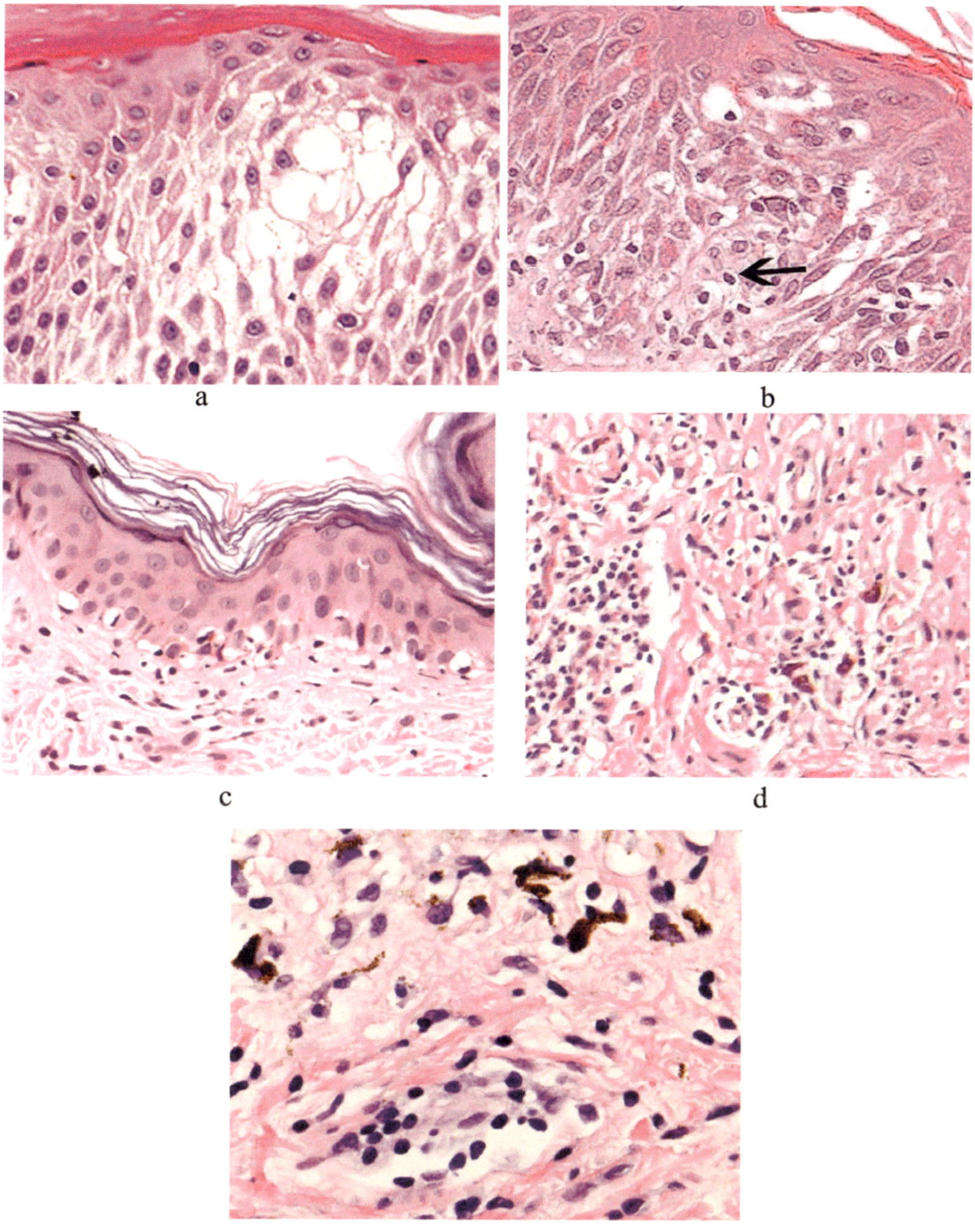

Figure 4.
(a) Spongiosis (H&E, x400). (b) Intraepidermal lymphocytes (H&E, x400). (c) Basal cell vacuolation (H&E, x400). (d) Dermal lymphocytosis (H&E, x200). (e) Dermal melanophages (H&E, x400).

features are not fully established. In a study carried out by the author, a reliable and systematic approach towards this diagnostic challenge has come up [49]. In that study the biopsies (3-mm punch) were taken from the margin of the active lesion.

The author recommends that while evaluating biopsies from cases of vitiligo histopathological examination should be primarily focused on evaluating five histopathological variables—spongiosis, epidermal lymphocytes, basal cell vacuolation, dermal lymphocytes and melanophages (**Figure 4**). The morphological criteria used to assess these parameters are listed in **Table 1**. All the cases are then scored

S. no.	Histological feature	Criteria
1	Spongiosis	Presence of at least one focus showing intercellular oedema in the epidermis
2	Epidermal lymphocytes	Presence of at least one lymphocyte in the epidermis
3	Basal cell vacuolation	Presence of at least one focus showing basal cell degeneration in the form of vacuolation
4	Melanophages	Presence of at least one focus in the superficial reticular dermis showing melanophages

Table 1.
Histomorphological criteria for spongiosis, epidermal lymphocytes, basal cell vacuolation and melanophages.

S. no.	Histological feature	Observation	Score
1	Spongiosis	Present/absent	1/0
2	Epidermal lymphocytes	Present/absent	1/0
3	Basal vacuolation	Present/absent	1/0
4	Dermal lymphocytes >100	Present/absent	1/0
5	Melanophages	Present/absence	1/0

Table 2.
Vitiligo histological scoring system.

S. no.	Total score	Diagnosis
1.	5	Unstable vitiligo
2.	4	Unstable vitiligo
3.	3	Favours unstable, clinical correlation required
4.	2	Favours stable, clinical correlation required
5.	0–1	Strongly favours stable vitiligo, clinical correlation essential

Table 3.
Final recommended diagnostic categories based on score.

using a scoring system devised by the authors **Table 2**, and the recommended diagnoses based on these scores are shown in **Table 3**. The counting for dermal lymphocytes was done in high power (x400) of a Nikon microscope. The scoring system can be applied to both segmental and non-segmental vitiligo. Adoption of a systematic reporting system brings more consistency and objectivity in the diagnosis.

4. Conclusions

Vitiligo is a common skin disorder which is characterized by the presence of depigmented milky white macules of variable sizes. Although there are various theories on its etiopathogenesis, the consensus opinion is that vitiligo occurs due to convergence various pathways. The basic histopathological finding in vitiligo is the absence of functional melanocytes in the basal layer of the epidermis. However, in order to evaluate for stability, the histopathological examination should be primarily focused on evaluating spongiosis, epidermal lymphocytes, basal cell vacuolation, dermal lymphocytes and melanophages. It is recommended to score these parameters, and the final report should incorporate recommended diagnosis based on the score. This will bring more objectivity and consistency in reporting these biopsies.

Acknowledgements

The author wishes to acknowledge the help provided by Dr. Niti Khunger, Consultant, Dermatology, VMMC & Safdarjung Hospital, and Dr. Pallavi Mishra, Resident, VMMC & Safdarjung Hospital.

Conflict of interest

The author wishes to declare that there are no conflicts of interest.

Notes/thanks/other declarations

None declared.

Author details

Amit Kumar Yadav
Department of Pathology, Vardhman Mahavir Medical College and Safdarjung Hospital, New Delhi, India

*Address all correspondence to: path.yadav@gmail.com

References

[1] Koranne RV, Sachdeva KG. Vitiligo. International Journal of Dermatology. 1988;**27**:676-681

[2] Nordlund JJ, Lerner AB. Vitiligo: It is important. Archives of Dermatology. 1982;**118**:5-8

[3] Sharquie KE. Vitiligo. Clinical and Experimental Dermatology. 1984;**9**:117-126

[4] Handa S, Kaur I. Vitiligo: Clinical findings in 1436 patients. The Journal of Dermatology. 1999;**26**:653-657

[5] Namazi MR. Phenytoin as a novel anti-vitiligo weapon. Journal of Autoimmune Diseases. 2005;**2**:11

[6] Mantovani S, Garbelli S, Palermo B, et al. Molecular and functional bases of self-antigen recognition in long-term persistent melanocyte-specific CD8+ T cells in one vitiligo patient. The Journal of Investigative Dermatology. 2003;**121**:308-314

[7] Xia Q, Zhou WM, Liang YH, et al. MHC haplotypic association in Chinese Han patients with vitiligo. Journal of the European Academy of Dermatology and Venereology. 2006;**20**:941-946

[8] Daneshpazhooh M, Mostofizadeh GM, Behjati J, Akhyani M, Mahmoud Robati R. Anti-thyroid peroxidase antibody and vitiligo: A controlled study. BMC Dermatology. 2006;**6**:3

[9] Alkahateeb A, Fain PR, Thody A, Bennett DC, Spritz RA. Epidemiology of vitiligo and associated autoimmune disease in Caucasian probands and their families. Pigment Cell Research. 2003;**16**:208-214

[10] Manolache L, Benea V. Stress in patients with alopecia areata and vitiligo. Journal of the European Academy of Dermatology and Venereology. 2007;**21**:921-928

[11] Le Poole IC, Das PK, Van den Wijngaard RM, Bos JD, Westerhof W. Review of the etiopathomechanism of vitiligo: A convergence theory. Experimental Dermatology. 1993;**2**:145-153

[12] Lerner AB. Vitiligo. The Journal of Investigative Dermatology. 1959;**32**:285-310

[13] Wu CS, Yu HS, Chang HR, Yu CL, Yu CL, Wu BN. Cutaneous blood flow and adrenoceptor response increase in segmental-type vitiligo lesions. Journal of Dermatological Science. 2000;**23**:53-62

[14] Al'Abadie MS, Senior HJ, Bleehen SS, Gawkrodger DJ. Neuropeptide and neuronal marker studies in vitiligo. The British Journal of Dermatology. 1994;**131**:160-165

[15] Yehuda R, Brand S, Yang RK. Plasma neuropeptide Y concentrations in combat exposed veterans: Relationship to trauma exposure, recovery from PTSD, and coping. Biological Psychiatry. 2006;**59**:660-663

[16] Kemp EH, Emhemad S, Akhtar S, Watson PF, Gawkrodger DJ, Weetman AP. Autoantibodies against tyrosine hydroxylase in patients with non-segmental (generalised) vitiligo. Experimental Dermatology. 2011;**20**:35-40

[17] Harning R, Cui J, Bystryn JC. Relation between the incidence and level of pigment cell antibodies and disease activity in vitiligo. The Journal of Investigative Dermatology. 1991;**97**:1078-1080

[18] Ingordo V, Gentile C, Iannazzone SS, Cusano F, Naldi L. Vitiligo

and autoimmunity: An epidemiological study in a representative sample of young Italian males. Journal of the European Academy of Dermatology and Venereology. 2011;**25**:105-109

[19] Uncu S, Yaylı S, Bahadır S, Okten A, Alpay K. Relevance of autoimmune thyroiditis in children and adolescents with vitiligo. International Journal of Dermatology. 2011;**50**:175-179

[20] Le Poole IC, van den Wijngaard RM, Westerhof W, Das PK. Presence of T cells and macrophages in inflammatory vitiligo skin parallels melanocyte disappearance. The American Journal of Pathology. 1996;**148**:1219-1228

[21] Grimes PE, Morris R, Avaniss-Aghajani E, Soriano T, Meraz M, Metzger A. Topical tacrolimus therapy for vitiligo: Therapeutic responses and skin messenger RNA expression of proinflammatory cytokines. Journal of the American Academy of Dermatology. 2004;**51**:52-61

[22] Taher ZA, Lauzon G, Maguiness S, Dytoc MT. Analysis of interleukin-10 levels in lesions of vitiligo following treatment with topical tacrolimus. The British Journal of Dermatology. 2009;**161**:654-659

[23] Bassiouny DA, Shaker O. Role of interleukin-17 in the pathogenesis of vitiligo. Clinical and Experimental Dermatology. 2011;**36**:292-297

[24] Ines D, Sonia B, Riadh BM, Amel el G, Slaheddine M, Hamida T, et al. A comparative study of oxidant-antioxidant status in stable and active vitiligo patients. Archives of Dermatological Research. 2006;298(4):**147**-152

[25] Dammak I, Boudaya S, Ben Abdallah F, Turki H, Attia H, Hentati B. Antioxidant enzymes and lipid peroxidation at the tissue level in patients with stable and active vitiligo. International Journal of Dermatology. 2009;**48**:476-480

[26] Hasse S, Gibbons NC, Rokos H, Marles LK, Schallreuter KU. Perturbed 6-tetrahydrobiopterin recycling via decreased dihydropteridine reductase in vitiligo: More evidence for H2O2 stress. The Journal of Investigative Dermatology. 2004;**122**:307-313

[27] Shalbaf M, Gibbons NC, Wood JM, Maitland DJ, Rokos H, Elwary SM, et al. Presence of epidermal allantoin further supports oxidative stress in vitiligo. Experimental Dermatology. 2008;**17**:761-770

[28] Bagherani N, Yaghoobi R, Omidian M. Hypothesis: Zinc can be effective in treatment of vitiligo. Indian Journal of Dermatology. 2011;**56**:480-484

[29] Yaghoobi R, Omidian M, Bagherani N. Vitiligo: A review of the published work. The Journal of Dermatology. 2011;**38**:419-431

[30] Hale LP. Zinc alpha-2-glycoprotein regulates melanin production by normal and malignant melanocytes. The Journal of Investigative Dermatology. 2002;**119**:464-470

[31] Akbayir N, Gökdemir G, Mansur T, Sökmen M, Gündüz S, Alkim C, et al. Is there any relationship between hepatitis C virus and vitiligo? Journal of Clinical Gastroenterology. 2004;**38**:815-817

[32] Toker SC, Sarycaoglu H, Karadogan SK, Mistik R, Baskan EB, Tunaly b. Is there any relation between vitiligo and cytomegalovirus? Journal of the European Academy of Dermatology and Venereology. 2007;**21**:141-142

[33] Niamba P, Traoré A, Taïeb A. Vitiligo in a black patient associated with HIV infection and repigmentation under antiretroviral therapy. Annales de Dermatologie et de Vénéréologie. 2007;**134**:272-273

[34] Lee AY, Youm YH, Kim NH, Yang H, Choi WI. Keratinocytes in the depigmented epidermis of vitiligo are more vulnerable to trauma (suction) than keratinocytes in the normally pigmented epidermis, resulting in their apoptosis. The British Journal of Dermatology. 2004;**151**:995-1003

[35] Bondanza S, Maurelli R, Paterna P, Migliore E, Giacomo FD, Primavera G, et al. Keratinocyte cultures from involved skin in vitiligo patients show an impaired in vitro behaviour. Pigment Cell Research. 2007;**20**:288-300

[36] van den Wijngaard R, Wankowicz-Kalinska A, Le Poole C, Tigges B, Westerhof W, Das P. Local immune response in skin of generalized vitiligo patients. Destruction of melanocytes is associated with the prominent presence of CLA+ T cells at the perilesional site. Laboratory Investigation. 2000;**80**:1299-1309

[37] Boissy RE, Liu YY, Medrano EE, Nordlund JJ. Structural aberration of the rough endoplasmic reticulum and melanosome compartmentalization in long-term cultures of melanocytes from vitiligo patients. The Journal of Investigative Dermatology. 1991;**97**:395-404

[38] Gauthier Y, Cario Andre M, Taïeb A. A critical appraisal of vitiligo etiologic theories. Is melanocyte loss a melanocytorrhagy? Pigment Cell Research. 2003;**16**:322-332

[39] Halder RM, Chappell JL. Vitiligo update. Seminars in Cutaneous Medicine and Surgery. 2009;**28**:86-92

[40] Haass NK, Herlyn M. Normal human melanocyte homeostasis as a paradigm for understanding melanoma. The Journal of Investigative Dermatology. Symposium Proceedings. 2005;**10**:153-163

[41] Lee AY, Kim NH, Choi WI, Youm YH. Less keratinocyte-derived factors related to more keratinocyte apoptosis in depigmented than normally pigmented suction blistered epidermis may cause passive melanocyte death in vitiligo. The Journal of Investigative Dermatology. 2005;**124**:976-983

[42] Le Poole IC, Das PK. Microscopic changes in vitiligo. Clinics in Dermatology. 1997;**15**:863-873

[43] Le Poole IC, van den Wijngaard RM, Westerhof W, Dutrieux RP, Das PK. Presence or absence of melanocytes in vitiligo lesions: An immunohistochemical investigation. The Journal of Investigative Dermatology. 1993;**100**:816-822

[44] Kim YC, Kim YJ, Kang HY, Sohn S, Lee ES. Histopathologic features in vitiligo. The American Journal of Dermatopathology. 2008;**30**:112-116

[45] Alikhan A, Felsten LM, Daly M, Petronic-Rosic V. Vitiligo: A comprehensive overview Part I. Introduction, epidemiology, quality of life, diagnosis, differential diagnosis, associations, histopathology, etiology, and work-up. Journal of the American Academy of Dermatology. 2011;**65**:473-491

[46] Wańkowicz-Kalińska A, van den Wijngaard RM, Tigges BJ, Westerhof W, Ogg GS, Cerundolo V, et al. Immunopolarization of CD4+ and CD8+ T cells to Type-1-like is associated with melanocyte loss in human vitiligo. Laboratory Investigation. 2003;**83**:683-695

[47] Boissy RE, Dell'Anna ML, Picardo M. On the pathophysiology of vitiligo: Possible treatment options. Indian Journal of Dermatology, Venereology and Leprology. 2012;**78**:24-29

[48] van den Boorn JG, Konijnenberg D, Dellemijn TA, van der Veen JP, Bos JD, Melief CJ, et al. Autoimmune destruction of skin melanocytes by perilesional T cells from vitiligo patients. The Journal of Investigative Dermatology. 2009;**129**:2220-2232

[49] Yadav AK, Singh P, Khunger N. Clinicopathologic analysis of stable and unstable vitiligo: A study of 66 cases. The American Journal of Dermatopathology. 2016;**38**(8):608-613

Chapter 4

Depigmentation's Disorders of the Vulva, Clinical Management

Panagiotis Tsikouras, Xanthoula Anthoulaki, Theodora Deftereou, Anastasia Bothou, Anna Chalkidou, Fotis Gasparos, Georgia Saradi, Dimitrios Tzeferakos, Elefterios Chatzimichael, Georgios Iatrakis, Stefanos Zervoudis and Georgios Galazios

Abstract

The cancer of the vulva is a rare disease with a positive association to poor developing countries. However, the incidence of vulvar cancer in situ nearly doubled in the last two decades and remained relatively stable. The main reason for this increased incidence of vulvar intraepithelial neoplasia (VIN) in women younger than 45 years is due to changes in sexual behavior, first intercourse at early age, multiple sexual partners, and sexually transmitted diseases that were increasing progressively. Furthermore, it is strongly associated with smoking and the increased incidence of HPV infection. The occurrence of early symptoms of VIN-like pruritus vulvae, pain, and lichen sclerosus led to early diagnosis to perform the adequate treatment. VIN tends to appear multifocal, while most invasive cancers are unilateral located and appeared with well-circumscribed lesions.

Keywords: lichen sclerosus vulvae, atrophic and hypertrophic disorders, vulvae, psoriasis

1. Introduction

1. The all vulva consisting of the mons pubis, the labia majora and minora, the clitoris, and the vulval vestibule, is covered by keratinized squamous epithelium as opposed to the vaginal mucosa covered by nonkeratinized epithelium of the same type. The labia majora carry hair and contain sebaceous and sweat glands. Embryologically, they correspond to the male scrotum. The lymph nodes of vulva drain to the external iliac lymph nodes via inguinal lymph nodes. The area is extremely vascular [1, 2].

2. After taking a detailed personal medical history regarding to hygiene techniques focusing on the use of antibiotic ointments, antiseptics, topical analgesics, lubricants should the gynecologist establish, whether the examining woman suffers from general skin conditions including dermatitis, psoriasis, lichen sclerosus, allergic contact dermatitis, or suspicious vulva disorders. It is commonly agreed that the rate of allergic dermatitis is high in combination to

IntechOpen

vulvar symptoms [3]. During the examination, the clinician should carefully examine the vulva and pay attention to skin or mucosal color (erythema and intense red); texture can provide clues to correct diagnosis (e.g., slight hyperkeratosis and thickened skin) existence of any lesions, which seems unusual for such macules, papules, or ulcers [4, 5]. Ulcers of vulva are diagnostically challenging due to variation in clinical morphology [4, 5]. The primary morphology is clinically relevant for identifying because it can significantly narrow the differential diagnosis. Diagnosis of vulvar ulcers based solely on clinical findings is often inaccurate, in most cases depending on sexually transmitted infections, but the differential diagnosis can include also dermatoses, trauma, neoplasms, hormonal-induced ulcers, drug reactions, or ulcer of unknown etiology [6, 7].

Subsequent to the completion of detailed observation, the clinician can decide for the diagnosis, if additional tools are necessary like speculum examination, vulvoscopy, or dermoscopy. The benefit of vulvoscopy remains controversial [8]. The contribution of dermoscope is mainly for the evaluation of both pigmented and nonpigmented lesions, presence of scarring, and loss of architecture but required training to identified benign structures and suspicious, worrisome features. It is crucial to document the number, type, size, border characteristics, and depth of lesions, discharge if present, tenderness, and presence or absence of local lymphadenopathy, which could influence mode of treatment [9, 10]. Cultures should be taken if there is suspicion for an infection, and final genital biopsies were recommended without to be prerequisite for the completion of the definitive diagnosis. It is an all common finding for a clinician to be frustrated by pathology report because it is sometimes difficult for the gynecologist due to inherent challenges to approach the obtaining tissue from the genitalia.

In 1976, Freidich classified skin disorders of the vulva into three categories: (a) hyperplastic dystrophy, (b) lichen sclerosus, and (c) dystrophy with or without atypia. For example, the term of hyperplastic dystrophy was used to include completely different clinical features, such as psoriasis, chronic lichen planus, and Bowen's disease [11].

Due to diagnostic problems resulting from this classification, in 1989, the International Society for the Study of Vulvar Diseases established a new terminology, which has been maintained to date [12]. Nonneoplastic epithelial lesions were delineated as follows: (a) lichen sclerosus and atrophicus, (b) squamous cell hyperplasia (former hyperplastic dystrophy without atypia), and (c) other diseases of vulva, a category in which various injuries occur, such as psoriasis, lichen planus, fungal infections, and condyloma acuminata. Since cytological atypia is found in this category, the damage is "changing" category and now belongs to the VIN classification [12].

2. Disorders of the vulva

2.1 Dermatopathies

"Dystrophy" of the vulva is an abnormality of the vulva epithelium. Epithelial growth may be hypoplastic, hyperplastic, or abnormal in some other way [13, 14].

2.1.1 Atrophic and hypertrophic disorders

Atrophic and hypertrophic disorders of the vulva come under the general term of dystrophies (formerly characterized as "precancerous" conditions). The skin, depending on the damage, may be appeared as white, dry, and thin or thickened, while hyperkeratosis and decreased vasculature are histologically present [15]. These alterations are mainly attributed to estrogen deficiency and, to this end, are often observed after menopause. The disorders may extend to the vaginal entrance, the perineum, etc. Usually there is intense pruritus, and the scratching it entails may result in an interception to the continuity of the skin. In addition to pruritus, there may be a burning sensation and dyspareunia, especially if the damage (usually atrophy) extends to the vaginal entrance [15]. For the treatment of pruritus, anti-inflammatory creams and topical corticosteroids are used (about two times a day). Antibiotic treatment is also administered in a transfection. In the absence of symptomatic treatment with conservative treatment and very intense annoyances of the patient, a simple vulvectomy can be chosen as "final" solution provided that the patient has been informed about the fact that in the half of the cases, the disease can relapse despite the surgical procedure [15].

Because of the fact that these disorders may coexist with malignancy, careful monitoring of the patient is required, and in doubt, multiple biopsies are required to exclude intraepithelial neoplasia (vulvar intraepithelial neoplasia/VIN) or cancer. Biopsies are often subjected to vulvovaginal screening after a 1–2% acetic acid solution is applied. However, the likelihood of developing invasive cancer in the soil of previous lesions is low. Given that these situations are well known, their descriptive "encyclopedic" terminology (in brackets, in italics) is not mentioned in the narrower "gynecological" or histological sense [16–21].

These alterations include:

- Lichen sclerosus
- Scuamous cell hyperplasia
- Condyloma acuminata
- Psoriasis
- Lichen planus
- Mixed lichen sclerosus and atrophicus

The term dystrophic lesions of the vulva according to literature like writhing, leukoplakia, lichen sclerosus and atrophicus, it is preferable to not be used anymore [16, 20, 21].

2.1.1.1 Lichen sclerosus

"Lichen sclerosus" (LS) is a term used for a benign, chronic, progressive dermatological condition characterized by (intense) inflammation [22–25]. The epithelium is getting thinner, and some characteristic dermatological changes appeared accompanied by itching and pain.

In general, lichen sclerosus appears in the skin of the genitalia. It was first described by Hallopeau and Darier at the end of the nineteenth century as a variety of lichen planus, which is not acceptable today. The term lichen sclerosus (and/or atrophicus) should no longer be used, as forms of lichen sclerosus are not all atrophic. When there is coexistence of squamous cell hyperplasia, it is characterized as "mixed squamous cell hyperplasia and lichen sclerosus" [26–32].

Lichen sclerosus is considered as the most common chronic lesion in vulva, referred to a chronic atrophy that usually observed after menopause. Clinically, vulva is glossy and dry, with no folds. The lesions are often symmetrical. Although the condition is observed over a wide range of ages, it has an increased incidence in women aged 50–59 years. Postmenopausal women and young girls are usually afflicted before menstruation. There is no clear justification. There is sufficient evidence of involvement of autoimmune mechanisms in the pathogenesis of lichen sclerosus. It is known that 21% of patients with lichen sclerosus also suffer from autoimmune disease more often than with thyroid disease. It is reported that 22% of patients with lichen sclerosus have an inherited history, and that 44% have one or more autoantibodies. Also, there is a correlation with HLA II antigens. There are studies associating inflammatory factors, e.g., Borrelia infection, with the development of lichen sclerosus. It is also reported that there is overexpression of wild-type P53 protein in lichen sclerosus, which occupies areas adjacent to squamous cell carcinoma (SCC) in which HPV is not detected.

Typically, the rash of lichen sclerosus begins as white polygonal papules, which flock to plaques. Typically, candlesticks and/or clearly cracked plugs appear on the surface of the plate, and they are similar to attached nozzles. Over time, plugs and craters may disappear by dropping a smooth, often porcelain plaque, and they rarely show up. Thus, the skin appears white and thin, although it may be present in SCH [26–32]. Originally, lichen sclerosus may have a bubbling consistency and is characterized by edema of the prepuce clitoris and telangiectasia of labia and purpura. Stretch marks appear mainly in the middle perineal line. Bullous lichen sclerosus is often accompanied by bleeding within the lesion, and the fillet can disappear. Later, labia minora and structures around clitoris disappeared too. The epithelium of the vagina and the cervix is not affected. However, there may be lesions in the forehead of the skin, which will lead to its constriction. Perianal lesions are described in 30% of cases [26–32].

Lichen sclerosus is a benign vulva condition associated to chronic and often progressive character with dermatologic location. Among the clinical findings are included marked inflammation, epithelial thinning, distinct dermal alterations like pruritus, and pain by varying degrees. The described lesions appear most frequently in the labia minora, but the early disease course affects not the vulvar architecture. During the disease progresses, the following pathological signs may be possible to occur: sexual dysfunction, fissuring in perineal region and around the clitoris, distinction between labia majora and minora, edema from inflammation, purpural lesions, and excoriations ecchymoses given fragility of the affected skin region [5, 33]. The main symptom is pruritus. Pain occurs if there are corrosions and stretch marks. Itching is intense during the night and may be so intense that it stops sleeping. Discomfort occurs when there is erosion, stretch marks, or narrowing of vaginal orifice [26–32]. Some women are asymptomatic, and LS is a random finding. Most of them had active childhood disease, which resulted in skin atrophy without symptomatology. Occasionally, hyperkeratosis and ecchymosis occur, which should be treated [26–32]. In childhood, the lesions are similar to adult lesions. But the ecchymosis may protrude and can be so intense that it leads us wrongly to the suspicion of sexual abuse. The diagnosis in most patients is indicated by the clinical picture, but its confirmation by histopathological examination is considered necessary. LS should be differentiated from lichen planus, vaginal pemphigoid, psoriasis, VIN, and SCC, and this is done by biopsy under colposcopic control. Ulcers, nodules, and granulomas should be controlled to exclude malignancy. The formation of hyperkeratotic plaques and erosions, which do not exist despite the applied treatment, suspects malignant transformation [26–32, 34].

Histologically, there is a decrease in subcutaneous fat, atrophy of all skin layers, and destruction of elastic tissue. The dermis is of some degree vitreous degeneration and round cell collections [35–37]. Typical histological findings are also including a thinned epidermis with areas hyperkeratosis, acanthosis, a broad band of homogenized collagen under the dermo-epidermal ligament, and lymphocyte infiltration under the homogenate area [33, 38–39].

Few patients have thickening of the epidermis, and these are those who have not been responding to LS and who are at increased risk of developing SCC. Due to the frequent association of LS with autoimmune diseases, the appropriate control should be performed. In particular, the possibility of autoimmune thyroid disease should be investigated [26–32, 34].

Squamous cell carcinoma (SCC) in women with LS is a common malignancy described. There are also reports of basal cell carcinoma and melanoma. The risk of developing SCC is about 5%. However, histopathologic examination in woman with lichen sclerosus during follow-up revealed squamous cell carcinoma. The role of HPV as a causative agent in malignant transformation is not entirely clear. There are studies suggesting the existence of two types of SCC: one type occurs in older patients with chronic LS disease and the other type is in younger women without LS but with proven infection by oncogenic HPV types. Although there is no evidence of the role of HPV as a causative agent in the development of SCC on LS, there is the theoretical risk of developing SCC from the topical use of corticosteroids, which may promote the development of HPV oncogenic strains, since it was found that in 20% of cases LS, there may be HPV infection [40–43]. More recent reports support the strong relationship of vulvar invasive squamous cell carcinoma and LS, so that lichen sclerosus is considered as precancerous damage [33]. It is not uncommon for women with carcinoma of vulva from squamous cells to also have undiagnosed lichen sclerosis, which may also be asymptomatic [33, 38].

The role of midwives, especially those who have increased initiatives due to their position (e.g., the one who works in the Center of Health), is very important to properly direct these postmenopausal women. It is well known that empirical use of ointments in precancerous or cancerous lesions of the vulva delays proper treatment and requires a high degree of suspicion of the doctor and midwife for malignant malignancy [33, 38].

There is no universally accepted treatment for women with lichen sclerosus. The treatment includes education and support, change of behavior to ensure good pudding hygiene, medication, and, in a small proportion of cases, surgery or photochemotherapy. The medical treatment of the condition includes the topical use of corticosteroids, such as clobetasol [44–47]. The major importance of LS treatment is proved by the fact that about 80% of invasive squamous cell carcinoma (SCC) of the vulva in elderly patients was associated with untreated, long-term conditions of lichen sclerosus (the final stage of the vicious cycle of itching-scratching-itching). Generally, the management should perform in twofold.

The first step aims to resolve LS symptoms, vulvar, and vaginal pain.

The second step's goal is to reduce the disease signs like hyperkeratosis fissuring echymoses [44–47].

2.1.1.2 Squamous cell hyperplasia

The oldest term leukoplakia ("chronic inflammatory disease of the mucosa which results in keratinization of the epithelium and in the formation of white spots") is still reported today. The disorder is characterized by white, tough, and overwhelmed, hyperkeratotic "plaques" of the vulvar epidermis, and a disorder of "hormonal homeostasis" in its etiology. Histologically, squamous cell hyperplasia is observed (**Figures 1** and **2**).

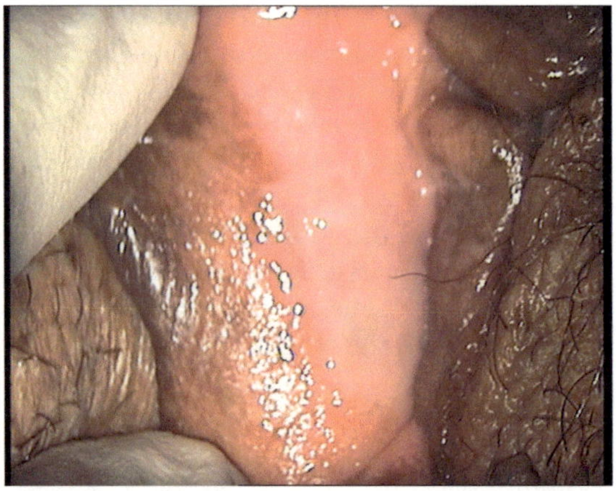

Figure 1.
VIN lesions are usually characterized by a change in color on the skin of the vulva. They are usually white and/or gray.

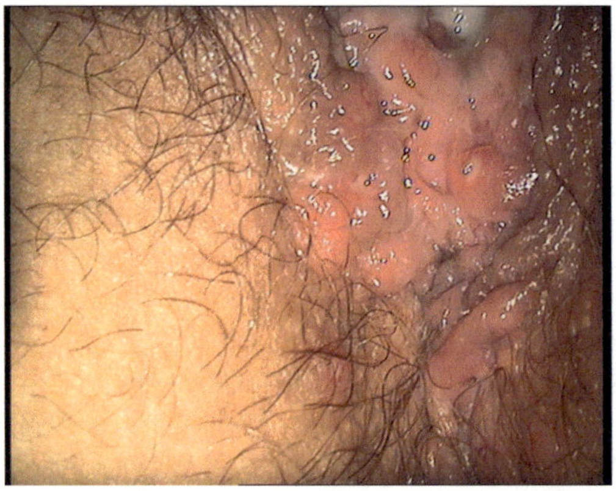

Figure 2.
VIN lesions: The rarities are lesions in red and brown. Their surface may be flat or abnormal.

This chronic and recurrent condition may occur at any age but is more common in older patients and usually manifests with pruritus. Less often, it occurs with dyspareunia or pain. It is an autoimmune condition and is associated with other autoimmune diseases such as malignant anemia, thyroid disease, diabetes mellitus, systemic lupus erythematosus, primary biliary cirrhosis, and bullous pemphigoid. Histologically, the skin appears thin with loss of the crevices found between the nipples. Surface skin is vitrified, and a set of chronic inflammatory cells is observed beneath it [48–53].

Clinically, the skin appears white, thin, and corrugated but may be overlapped and keratinized, if there is coexistence of squamous cell hyperplasia. There may also be symphysis of the clitoris or the vulva. The diagnosis is made by biopsy. Lichen sclerosus is a nonneoplastic condition but can coexist with vulvar intraepithelial neoplasia, while there is correlation with invasive squamous cell carcinoma of the vulva in 2–5% of cases. This is describing the reason why possible long-term monitoring is required every 6–12 months [26–32].

Treatment is required, especially if the condition is symptomatic, and a strong local topical steroid cream (e.g., Dermovate per 12-hour period) is usually used, which is gradually replaced by a milder formulation (e.g., hydrocortisone per hour, 24 h or less) as the symptoms require. Fluorinated corticosteroids or testosterone ointment may also be helpful. Vulvectomy has no position in this case, as the recurrence rate after surgery is about 50% [26–32].

2.1.1.3 Psoriasis

Psoriasis is manifested as dry, red, and papular rash, which is usually clearly circumscribed and extends to the thighs. Diagnosis occurs easily when bleeding is observed during the removal of classic silver-like scars. It may be difficult to differentiate psoriasis from candida infection or dermatitis because the vulva is very often fluid. Candida infection should be ruled out. The lesions can be treated locally with coal tar preparations, ultraviolet maize, steroid creams, or other suitable drugs [54–56].

2.1.1.4 Lichen planus

It is a chronic papular rash with a bluish hue, which is located in the vulva and the bendable surfaces. It may be appeared in other areas like the mucous membrane of the oral cavity, and the diagnosis is enhanced by finding other lesions. Oral lesions precede genital lesions in one-third and simultaneously appear in half of women affected from the disease. After the vulva should be a vaginal examination, the walls of the vaginal may have following pathological abnormalities: erythema erosions and bleeding friable tissue. It is usually idiopathic but can also be related to medications. The treatment includes use of strong steroids locally or ultraviolet light, and the disease tends to subside within the next 2 years. Surgery removal should be avoided [57–62].

2.1.2 Others: vitiligo, intertrigo, aphthae

2.1.2.1 Vitiligo

The lesions of this disease can appear anywhere on the body with a predilection in the genital area. It can be confused with LS, associated to lack the classical signs of inflammation, possible coexistence with LS based on autoimmunogenity. In contrast to LS, which has predilection for hypoostrogenic states, vitiligo can be appeared at any age. No skin biopsies are necessary. Autoimmune thyroid disease is associated to vitiligo. Treatment includes administration of topical steroids and vitamins D, E, C, and B12. Surgery remains a viable option in unresponsive localized disease to conventional therapies [63–71].

2.1.2.2 Apthtae

They are vulva disorder associated to pain. Shallow ulcers most commonly occur on the oral mucosa and less commonly on the genital mucosa. The reasons are uncertain, and risk factors include stress, infections, hormonal factors, vitamin deficiency, and family history. The diagnosis result from exclusion of various genital ulcers causing in most cases in assumption of sexually transmitted infection. Aphthosis appears in simple and rare complex form, and the recurrence rate is about 20% of the general population. For the treatment, it is important to educate the patients to conform in skin and wound care and administration of topical corticosteroid propionate ointment in cases of complex aphthosis [63–71]. Apthae should differentiate from Behcet syndrome, a disorder that causes inflammation of the blood vessels throughout the body, and could affect the vuvla causing open sores in the vulva. Furthermore, vulva aphthous ulcers could appear in patients with HIV infection, Chrohn disease, and ulcerative colitis.

2.1.2.3 Intertrigo combined with candida infection

Intertrigo is a wet inflammatory dermatitis, which can occur on any fold of the body because of the irritation of the exposed skin surfaces from friction between them. This is more likely to occur in women who are overweight but also in those who wear tight clothing.

The skin is painful, often red and flaky, showing wetness and stretch marks. Weight loss, local hygiene, and local exposure to air, such as the use of socks and cotton lingerie instead of synthetic underwear, should be envisioned. Powders (e.g., talc), astringents (e.g., zinc), or blocking agents in the area may also help.

Candida usually complicates intertrigo and should be treated as described according to clinical practice guidelines for the management of candidiasis [56, 57]. In order to relief the inflammation, since there is no candida infection, steroid creams may be used.

2.1.3 Allergic/irritant dermatitis

The skin of the vulva, and especially the opening of vagina, is often affected by dermatitis. Dermatitis can be irritating (nonimmune) or actually allergic (immune-induced). Chemicals that cause skin hypersensitivity include, but are not limited to, cosmetics, perfumes, contraceptive lubricants, sprays, and vaginal washings. Detergents, dyes, softeners, bleaches, soaps, and bleach used to clean the underwear can also cause irritation. In severe cases, hypersensitivity may occur in topical application of anesthetic creams, as well as steroid preparations.

Women with contact dermatitis have an overgrowth inflamed vulva with eczema characters, and patch tests can reveal local irritants. Temporary relief can be achieved with lubricants of the vulva (e.g., Emulsiderm in a daily bath), softeners (e.g., local water creams), and topical corticosteroids (e.g., monthly treatment with Dermovate topical application). As before, nonresponsive lesions need biopsy to confirm the diagnosis [72–75].

2.2 Pruritus

The term pruritus describes an intense feeling of itching. It is more common in women over the age of 40 years, and symptoms are getting worse by stress or depression. There are many causes of itching.

Biopsy may be necessary for diagnosis, as well as patch tests may be also helpful. If no cause is found, it may be worth considering the possibility of previous sexual abuse or psychosocial problems.

It is important to stop the vicious cycle of irritation/itching cycle that is using strong local steroids for a short time in order to reduce the local inflammation induced by scratching. Applying strong steroid ointment daily for 3 weeks followed by 1% hydrocortisone cream once a day is useful, as well as soap substitutes (e.g., Oilatum).

Irritants, cosmetics added to bath, and synthetic pantyhose, as well as soap substitutes, should be avoided, and comfortable cotton underwear should be used. The area should be gently dry (e.g., with a hairdryer). Antihistamines can also help. If depression coexists, it may require treatment [76–84].Reasons of vaginal pruritus

Infection (candida, luteum, filamentous worms)
Eczema
Dermatitis (patch tests)
Irritation due to vaginal excretion
Lichen sclerosus
Lichen planus

Vulvar intraepithelial neoplasia (VIN)
Vulvar cancer
Systematic diseases (diabetes mellitus, ureamia, or liver deficiency)
Psychogenic [82–84]

2.3 Vulvar intraepithelial neoplasia (VIN)

The term VIN was proposed to include dysplastic lesions and vulvar squamous in situ cancer and replace terms such as: (a) Bowen's disease; (b) Bowen's papilloma; and (c) dystrophy with atypia.

Depending on the degree of maturation of the neoplastic epithelium and the extent of atypia, three VIN classes, from I to III, are defined just like in CIN.

2.3.1 New terminology: previous terminology

VIN I: mild dysplasia
VIN II: moderate dysplasia
VIN III: Toy Bowen's disease, severe dysplasia
Squamous cell carcinoma in situ, erythroplasia of Queyrat

The lesion is characterized as VIN I when the cellular abnormalities, in comparison with absence of layout, are limited to the lower one-third of the vulvar squamous epithelium, VIN II when the abnormalities extend to the middle third of the epithelium, VIN III when they extend to the upper third of the epithelium, and CIS when lesions occupy all the epithelial layers. Approximately 40% of women present without accompanied symptoms and in the rest cases a background of inflammatory skin disease in the majority being lichen sclerosus exist.

The disease is not characterized as invasive carcinoma as long as the basal lamina remains intact [72–75].

2.3.2 Risk factors VIN

Common point: VIN is part of a total of epithelial changes in the woman's inferior genital system and may coexist (at least 15–20%). In particular, if there are acuminate warts in the vulva, the rate for CIN lesions is almost 50%.

2.3.3 Risk factors

1. Early onset of sexual activity
2. Switching (multiple) sexual partners
3. Immune system weakness
4. Cross-reaction or coexistence of high-risk HPV subtypes
5. Smoking, alcohol, and unbalanced diet
6. HPV infection
7. HSV-2 infection
8. Chronic irritation of the vulva
9. Warts

2.3.4 Biological behavior and prognosis VIN and CIN

In most VIN cases, instead of CIN, the damage is high risk. It is also uncommon to diagnose just VIN I lesion.

VIN:

- increased incidence in last two decades
- average age of development 30 years
- risk of progression to invasive cancer increased in women of the fifth decade (20%)
- the recession is twice as likely as invasion.

It is more common in women of 20–30 years, while VIN III in the fourth decade whereas invasive cancer mainly in the fifth decade [32, 34, 40].

2.3.5 Clinical finding and diagnose of VIN and CIN

VIN instead of CIN is not appeared during colposcopy with abnormal vasculation and mosaicism, but in the form of subtracted white or red plaques with clear borders.

Due to keratinization of the surface layer, in case of VIN, the cytological evaluation is more difficult.

VIN: itching, burning sensation, pain, single, or multifocal lesions (40%)
CIN: there are usually no symptoms or findings, single, or multifocal lesions
VIN: lesions often situated in the inner lips of vagina and the perineum
CIN: lesions frequently cited in the transformation zone

3 Basic principles in treatment of depigmentation disorders of the vulva

3.1 Clobetazole (Butavate*)

Treatment of choice is the topical administration of clobetazole, which blocks mitosis and induces synthesis of proteins reducing inflammatory response. It is also believed that it affects Ki67 as well as promotes p53 expression.

For those cases that diagnosed for the first time, it is recommended to apply once daily for 4 weeks, then every second day for 4 more weeks and during the third month of treatment, twice a week (once a day is based on pharmacokinetic studies). If symptoms reappear, the minimal clobetazole dose in which disease was controlled is administered.

A 30 g tube should be used for 12 weeks, and then, the original is reconsidered. If treatment is effective, hyperkeratosis, bruising, erosions, and stretch marks will disappear, but atrophy and color change still remain.

Clobetazole is continued as needed. Most patients usually need 30–60 g per year. If therapy is complete, no further treatment is needed, but other patients will have relapses and should continue to receive treatment [72–75].

An alternative option is triamcinolone ointments.

3.2 Testosterone and other hormones

Nowadays, estrogens or testosterone creams have no place in the LS treatment. Also recent studies have shown that testosterone is less effective than clobetazole and has same effectiveness with petrolatum, the excipient used to make testosterone ointment.

3.3 Progesterone

It is referred to be extremely effective. It is prepared by mixing 400 mg progesterone oil with 4 oz Aqua-for. It is prescribed twice a day.

3.4 Retinoids

They are mainly used in the complicated LS on failure of corticoid treatment. It is considered that they reduce the degradation of the connective tissue.

3.4.1 Acitrecine (Nco-Tigason)*

Acitrecine (Nco-Tigason*) 25 or 50 mg/24 h per os in a single dose until symptom remission and continue 25–50 mg/24 hours go per os. The treatment stops when the lesions fall back.

3.4.2 Isotretinoin (Roaccutan, Accurane*)*

Isotretinoin (Roaccutan*, Accurane*) synthetic 13 is isomer of tretinoin. It reduces sebaceous gland size and sebum production and inhibits abnormal keratinization. The dose is 0.5–1 mg/kg/24 hours, and the duration of treatment is 4–6 months.

Topical administration of retinoids is not recommended due to the local irritation they cause.

Close attention should be paid to per os administration of retinoids to adolescents due to the teratogenicity they cause and is recommended avoidance of pregnancy for 2 months (isotretinoin) and 3 years (acitretin) at the end of the treatment [72–75].

3.5 Other medications

Positive results from the administration of potassium para-aminobenzoate, as well as psoralen with UVA therapy, stanozolol, antimalarials, antihistamines (e.g. oxatomide), and various antibiotics (possible cause or infection by Borrelia), were also observed.

3.6 Surgical treatment

In uncomplicated forms of LS, there is no evidence of removal of vulvar tissue. Surgical treatment should be applied exclusively in case of malignant transformation and recurrent forms.

When there is a narrowing of the opening of vagina, perineoplasty is performed, which improves dyspareunia in 90% of cases and improves the quality of sexual life in 86% of cases.

Simple vulvectomy should not be preferred because the symptoms do not always disappear, the signs reappear, and the likelihood of malignant transformation persists. Also, the operation creates many psychosocial problems.

3.7 Alternative treatment

Positive results are reported with LASER ablation treatment, which is applied with LASER CO, 1–2 mm deep with complete healing 6 weeks after surgery and low relapse rates. It is considered a method of nonresponse to other forms of treatment.

Photodynamic therapy (topical application of the 5-aminolevulinic acid photosensitizer and exposure to argon laser light for 1–2 alphas in 1–3 sessions) is also used with very good results.

3.8 General considerations for patients during treatment

Patients with LS have thin skin, which is not considered a "satisfactory" barrier to the loss of moisture, and it would be a failure not to mention some general measures.

1. Excessive drying after bathing should be avoided.

2. Gentle moisturizing products such as, e.g., Vaseline should be used to improve the moisture of the affected skin.

3. Good hygiene, avoidance of irritants and allergens, use of cotton lingerie, and avoidance of tight and hot clothes.

A lesion that resides in the vulva or in the vaginal opening and continues after the skin lesion is absent is secondary to a sensory disorder. This pain does not correspond to topical administration of corticosteroids. A 5% xylocaine ointment is therapeutically administered; on failure, administration of amitriptyline is recommended [72–75].

3.9 Failure of treatment

On unsuccessful treatment with corticosteroids, the following should be checked: patient compliance, misdiagnosis or coexistence of other disease entities, contact dermatitis, secondary candidiasis, VIN, SCC, psoriasis, or pemphigoid vulgaris.

If the symptoms persist after the medical repair of the damage, it is a secondary sensory disorder.

3.10 Follow-up

The risk of malignant transformation of LS is very small. Even if malignant transformation occurs, the progression of the disease is slow. However, patients should be screened at the end of the first trimester of treatment after 6 months and then yearly.

One-month follow-up requires patients with a poor response to corticosteroid therapy, and they are usually those in whom squamous cell hyperplasia coexists and are therefore susceptible to malignant transformation.

4. Conclusion

Vulva pathology is varied. Between all the described lesions, precancer conditions should be recognized early in order to stop the evolution. Strong dermocorticoids are the major local treatment on many vulvae chronic diseases. In specific conditions, local immune modulators or laser are necessary.

Acknowledgements

Many thanks to midwives (Mrs. Maria Strofali and Mrs. Stavroula Falaga) of family planning center, Democritus University of Thrace, Greece for their clinical support and examination of women, who visited our family planning examination center.

Author details

Panagiotis Tsikouras[1*], Xanthoula Anthoulaki[1], Theodora Deftereou[1], Anastasia Bothou[1], Anna Chalkidou[1], Fotis Gasparos[2], Georgia Saradi[2], Dimitrios Tzeferakos[2], Elefterios Chatzimichael[1], Georgios Iatrakis[3], Stefanos Zervoudis[2] and Georgios Galazios[1]

1 Department of Obstetrics and Gynecology, Democritus University of Thrace, Greece

2 Department of Obstetrics and Gynecology, Rea Hospital, Athens, Greece

3 Department of Obstetrics and Gynecology, University of West Attica, Greece

*Address all correspondence to: ptsikour@med.duth.gr

References

[1] Cohen Sacher B. The normal vulva, vulvar examination, and evaluation tools. Clinical Obstetrics and Gynecology. 2015;**58**(3):442-452. DOI: 10.1097/GRF.0000000000000123

[2] Basaran M, Kosif R, Bayar U, Civelek B. Characteristics of external genitalia in pre- and postmenopausal women. Climacteric. 2008;**11**(5):416-421. DOI: 10.1080/13697130802366670

[3] Woodruff CM, Trivedi MK, Botto N, Kornik R. Allergic contact dermatitis of the vulva. Dermatitis. 2018;**29**(5):233-243

[4] Lloyd J, Crouch NS, Minto CL, Liao LM, Creighton SM. Female genital appearance: "Normality" unfolds. BJOG: An International Journal of Obstetrics and Gynaecology. 2005;**112**(5):643-646

[5] Howarth H, Sommer V, Jordan FM. Visual depictions of female genitalia differ depending on source. Medical Humanities. 2010;**36**(2):75-79. DOI: 10.1136/jmh.2009.003707

[6] Covino JM, McCormack WM. Vulvar ulcer of unknown etiology in a human immunodeficiency virus-infected woman: Response to treatment with zidovudine. American Journal of Obstetrics and Gynecology. 1990;**163** (1 Pt 1):116-118

[7] Micheletti L, Bogliatto F, Lynch PJ, Bandow GD. Diagnosis and management of vulvar ulcers. Dermatologic Clinics. 2010;**28**(4):753-763. DOI: 10.1016/j.det.2010.08.008

[8] Micheletti L, Bogliatto F, Lynch PJ. Vulvoscopy: Review of a diagnostic approach requiring clarification. The Journal of Reproductive Medicine. 2008;**53**(3):179-182

[9] Stecklein SR, Frumovitz M, Klopp AH, Gunther JR, Eifel PJ. Effectiveness of definitive radiotherapy for squamous cell carcinoma of the vulva with gross inguinal lymphadenopathy. Gynecologic Oncology. 2018;**148**(3):474-479

[10] Eva LJ. Screening and follow up of vulval skin disorders. Best Practice & Research. Clinical Obstetrics & Gynaecology. 2012;**26**(2):175-188. DOI: 10.1016/j.bpobgyn.2011.11.005

[11] Freidrich EG Jr. Vulvar disease. Major Problems in Obstetrics and Gynecology. 1976;**9**:1-217

[12] Ridley CM, Frankman O, Jones IS, Pincus SH, Wilkinson EJ, Fox H, et al. New nomenclature for vulvar disease: International society for the study of vulvar disease. Human Pathology. 1989;**20**(5):495-496

[13] Rodriguez MI, Leclair CM. Benign vulvar dermatoses. Obstetrical & Gynecological Survey. 2012;**67**(1):55-63. DOI: 10.1097/OGX.0b013e318240cc72

[14] Simonetta C, Burns EK, Guo MA. Vulvar dermatoses: A review and update. Missouri Medicine. 2015;**112**(4):301-307

[15] Farage MA, Miller KW, Ledger WJ. Determining the cause of vulvovaginal symptoms. Obstetrical & Gynecological Survey. 2008;**63**(7):445-464. DOI: 10.1097/OGX.0b013e318172ee25

[16] Stockdale CK, Boardman L. Diagnosis and treatment of vulvar dermatoses. Obstetrics and Gynecology. 2018;**131**(2):371-386. DOI: 10.1097/AOG.0000000000002460

[17] Belotto RA, Chavantes MC, Tardivo JP, Euzébio Dos Santos R, Fernandes RCM, et al. Therapeutic comparison between treatments for vulvar lichen sclerosus: Study protocol of a randomized prospective

and controlled trial. BMC Women's Health. 2017;**17**(1):61. DOI: 10.1186/s12905-017-0414-y

[18] Sideri M, Jones RW, Wilkinson EJ, Preti M, Heller DS, Scurry J, et al. Squamous vulvar intraepithelial neoplasia: 2004 modified terminology, ISSVD vulvar oncology subcommittee. The Journal of Reproductive Medicine. 2005;**50**(11):807-810

[19] Committee on Gynecologic Practice of American College Obstetricians and Gynecologists ACOG. Committee opinion No. 509: Management of vulvar intraepithelial neoplasia. Obstetrics and Gynecology. 2011;**118**(5):1192-1194. DOI: 10.1097/AOG.0b013e31823b17c2

[20] Bornstein J, Goldstein AT, Stockdale CK, Bergeron S, Pukall C, Zolnoun D, et al. 2015 ISSVD, ISSWSH, and IPPS consensus terminology and classification of persistent vulvar pain and vulvodynia. Consensus vulvar pain terminology committee of the International Society for the Study of vulvovaginal disease (ISSVD), the International Society for the Study of Women's sexual health (ISSWSH), and the international pelvic pain society (IPPS). Journal of Lower Genital Tract Disease. 2016;**20**(2):126-130. DOI: 10.1097/LGT.0000000000000019

[21] Bornstein J, Bogliatto F, Haefner HK, Stockdale CK, Preti M, Bohl TG, et al. The 2015 International Society for the Study of vulvovaginal disease (ISSVD) terminology of vulvar squamous intraepithelial lesions. Obstetrics and Gynecology. 2016;**127**(2):264-268. DOI: 10.1097/AOG.0000000000001285

[22] Ball SB, Wojnarowska F. Vulvar dermatoses: Lichen sclerosus, lichen planus, and vulval dermatitis/lichen simplex chronicus. Seminars in Cutaneous Medicine and Surgery. 1998;**17**(3):182-188

[23] Zendell K, Edwards L. Lichen sclerosus with vaginal involvement: Report of 2 cases and review of the literature. JAMA Dermatology. 2013;**149**(10):1199-1202. DOI: 10.1001/jamadermatol.2013.4885

[24] Funaro D. Lichen sclerosus: A review and practical approach. Dermatologic Therapy. 2004;**17**(1):28-37

[25] Haefner HK, Aldrich NZ, Dalton VK, Gagné HM, Marcus SB, Patel DA, et al. The impact of vulvar lichen sclerosus on sexual dysfunction. Journal of Women's Health (2002). 2014;**23**(9):765-770. DOI: 10.1089/jwh.2014.4805

[26] Moyal-Barracco M, Wendling J. Vulvar dermatosis. Best Practice & Research. Clinical Obstetrics & Gynaecology. 2014;**28**(7):946-958. DOI: 10.1016/j.bpobgyn.2014.07.005

[27] Heller DS. Benign papular lesions of the vulva. Journal of Lower Genital Tract Disease. 2012;**16**(3):296-305. DOI: 10.1097/LGT.0b013e31823f4323. Review

[28] Fite C, Plantier F, Dupin N, Avril MF, Moyal-Barracco M. Vulvar verruciform xanthoma: Ten cases associated with lichen sclerosus, lichen planus, or other conditions. Archives of Dermatology. 2011;**147**(9):1087-1092. DOI: 10.1001/archdermatol.2011.113

[29] Kelekci KH, Adamhasan F, Gencdal S, Sayar H, Kelekci S. The impact of the latest classification system of benign vulvar diseases on the management of women with chronic vulvar pruritus. Indian Journal of Dermatology, Venereology and Leprology. 2011;**77**(3):294-299. DOI: 10.4103/0378-6323.79698

[30] Papalas JA, Sangueza OP, Puri PK, Robboy SJ, Selim MA. Vulvar vascular tumors: A clinicopathologic study of 85 patients. The American Journal of Dermatopathology.

2013;**35**(1):1-7; quiz 8-10. DOI: 10.1097/DAD.0b013e31823135c5

[31] Mayeaux EJ Jr, Cooper D. Vulvar procedures: Biopsy, bartholin abscess treatment, and condyloma treatment. Obstetrics and Gynecology Clinics of North America. 2013;**40**(4):759-772

[32] Larrabee R, Kylander DJ. Benign vulvar disorders. Identifying features, practical management of nonneoplastic conditions and tumors. Postgraduate Medicine. 2001;**109**(5):151, 4, 157-159, 163-164

[33] Regauer S, Liegl B, Reich O, Pickel H, Beham-Schmid C. Vulvar lichen sclerosus. The importance of early clinical and histological diagnosis. Der Hautarzt. 2004;**55**(2):158-164

[34] Fistarol SK, Itin PH. Anti-inflammatory treatment. Current Problems in Dermatology. 2011;**40**: 58-70. DOI: 10.1159/000321051

[35] Karadag AS, Kavala M, Ozlu E, Zindancı İ, Ozkanlı S, Turkoglu Z, et al. The co-occurrence of lichen sclerosus et atrophicus and celiac disease. Indian Dermatology Online Journal. 2014;**5**(Suppl 2):S106-S108. DOI: 10.4103/2229-5178.146172

[36] Fistarol SK, Itin PH. Diagnosis and treatment of lichen sclerosus: An update. American Journal of Clinical Dermatology. 2013;**14**(1):27-47. DOI: 10.1007/s40257-012-0006-4

[37] Lee A, Bradford J, Fischer G. Long-term management of adult vulvar lichen sclerosus: A prospective cohort study of 507 women. JAMA Dermatology. 2015;**151**(10):1061-1067. DOI: 10.1001/jamadermatol.2015.0643

[38] Chibnall R. Vulvar pruritus and lichen simplex chronicus. Obstetrics and Gynecology Clinics of North America. 2017;**44**(3):379-388. DOI: 10.1016/j.ogc.2017.04.003

[39] Rotsztejn H. Some remarks about lichen sclerosus vulvae. Ginekologia Polska. 2004;**75**(12):979-983

[40] Handisurya A, Schellenbacher C, Kirnbauer R. Diseases caused by human papillomaviruses (HPV). Journal der Deutschen Dermatologischen Gesellschaft. 2009;**7**(5):453, 467-66; quiz 466. DOI: 10.1111/j.1610-0387.2009.06988.x

[41] Ljubojević S, Lipozencić J, Skerlev M, Zele-Starcević L, Ljubojević N, Babić D, et al. Diagnostic-therapeutic guidelines for men whose partners have HPV genital infection. Liječnički Vjesnik. 2009;**131**(9-10):269-274

[42] Ljubojević S, Lipozencić J, Grgec DL, Prstacić R, Skerlev M, Mokos ZB. Human papilloma virus associated with genital infection. Collegium Antropologicum. 2008;**32**(3):989-997. Review

[43] Ljubojevic S, Skerlev M. HPV-associated diseases. Clinics in Dermatology. 2014;**32**(2):227-234. DOI: 10.1016/j.clindermatol.2013.08.007

[44] Schlosser BJ, Mirowski GW. Lichen sclerosus and lichen planus in women and girls. Clinical Obstetrics and Gynecology. 2015;**58**(1):125-142. DOI: 10.1097/GRF.0000000000000090

[45] Thorstensen KA, Birenbaum DL. Recognition and management of vulvar dermatologic conditions: Lichen sclerosus, lichen planus, and lichen simplex chronicus. Journal of Midwifery & Women's Health. 2012;**57**(3):260-275. DOI: 10.1111/j.1542-2011.2012.00175.x

[46] Marnach ML, Torgerson RR. Vulvovaginal issues in mature women. Mayo Clinic Proceedings. 2017;**92**(3):449-454. DOI: 10.1016/j.mayocp.2016.10.031

[47] Pérez-López FR, Vieira-Baptista P. Lichen sclerosus in women: A review.

Climacteric. 2017;**20**(4):339-347. DOI: 10.1080/13697137.2017.1343295

[48] Guerrero A, Venkatesan A. Inflammatory vulvar dermatoses. Clinical Obstetrics and Gynecology. 2015;**58**(3):464-475. DOI: 10.1097/GRF.0000000000000125

[49] Barchino-Ortiz L, Suárez-Fernández R, Lázaro-Ochaita P. Vulvar inflammatory dermatoses. Actas Dermo-Sifiliográficas. 2012;**103**(4):260-275. DOI: 10.1016/j.ad.2011.08.001

[50] O'Connell TX, Nathan LS, Satmary WA, Goldstein AT. Non-neoplastic epithelial disorders of the vulva. American Family Physician. 2008;**77**(3):321-326

[51] Heller DS. Benign tumors and tumor-like lesions of the vulva. Clinical Obstetrics and Gynecology. 2015;**58**(3):526-535. DOI: 10.1097/GRF.0000000000000133

[52] Allbritton JI. Vulvar neoplasms, benign and malignant. Obstetrics and Gynecology Clinics of North America. 2017;**44**(3):339-352. DOI: 10.1016/j.ogc.2017.04.002

[53] Ganovska A, Kovachev S. Vulvar intraepithelial neoplasia–Terminology, symptoms and treatment. Akush Ginekol (Sofiia). 2015;**54**(7):36-40

[54] Sand FL, Thomsen SF. Skin diseases of the vulva: Eczematous diseases and contact urticaria. Journal of Obstetrics and Gynaecology. 2018;**38**(3):295-300. DOI: 10.1080/01443615.2017.1329283

[55] Crone AM, Stewart EJ, Wojnarowska F, Powell SM. Aetiological factors in vulvar dermatitis. Journal of the European Academy of Dermatology and Venereology. 2000

[56] Blostein F, Levin-Sparenberg E, Wagner J, Foxman B. Recurrent vulvovaginal candidiasis. Annals of Epidemiology. 2017;**27**(9):575-582.e3. DOI: 10.1016/j.annepidem.2017.08.010

[57] Pappas PG, Kauffman CA, Andes D, Benjamin DK Jr, Calandra TF, Edwards JE Jr, et al. Clinical practice guidelines for the management of candidiasis: 2009 update by the Infectious Diseases Society of America. Clinical Infectious Diseases. 2009;**48**(5):503-535. DOI: 10.1086/596757

[58] van de Nieuwenhof HP, Bulten J, Hollema H, Dommerholt RG, Massuger LF, van der Zee AG, et al. Differentiated vulvar intraepithelial neoplasia is often found in lesions, previously diagnosed as lichen sclerosus, which have progressed to vulvar squamous cell carcinoma. Modern Pathology. 2011;**24**(2):297-305. DOI: 10.1038/modpathol.2010.192

[59] Goldnau C, Köninger A, Kimmig R. The female external genitalia: Pathologic findings and first steps in treatment. Urologe A. 2010;**49**(12):1496-1502. DOI: 10.1007/s00120-010-2407-4

[60] Roh MR, Choi YJ, Lee KG. Papular acantholytic dyskeratosis of the vulva. The Journal of Dermatology. 2009;**36**(7):427-429. DOI: 10.1111/j.1346-8138.2009.00660.x

[61] Bauer A, Rodiger C, Greif C, Kaatz M, Elsner P. Vulvar dermatoses–Irritant and allergic contact dermatitis of the vulva. Dermatology. 2005;**210**(2):143-149

[62] Sand FL, Thomsen SF. Skin diseases of the vulva: Eczematous diseases and contact urticarial. Journal of Obstetrics and Gynaecology. 2018;**38**(3):295-300. DOI: 10.1080/01443615.2017.1329283

[63] Hengge UR, Meurer M. Pigmented lesions of the genital mucosa. Der Hautarzt. 2005;**56**(6):540-549

[64] O'Donnell AT, Kim CC. Update and clinical use of imaging technologies for

pigmented lesions of the skin. Seminars in Cutaneous Medicine and Surgery. 2012;**31**(1):38-44. DOI: 10.1016/j.sder.2011.12.003

[65] Collas H, Delbarre M, De Preville PA, Courville P, Neveu C, Dompmartin A, et al. Evaluation of the diagnosis of pigmented tumors of the skin and factors leading to a decision to excise. Dermatologists of the postgraduate Association of Haute-Normandie. Annales de Dermatologie et de Vénéréologie. 1999;**126**(6-7):494-500

[66] Ronger-Savle S, Julien V, Duru G, Raudrant D, Dalle S, Thomas L. Features of pigmented vulval lesions on dermoscopy. The British Journal of Dermatology. 2011;**164**(1):54-61. DOI: 10.1111/j.1365-2133.2010.10043.x

[67] Edwards L. Pigmented vulvar lesions. Dermatologic Therapy. 2010;**23**(5):449-457. DOI: 10.1111/j.1529-8019.2010.01349.x

[68] Venkatesan A. Pigmented lesions of the vulva. Dermatologic Clinics. 2010;**28**(4):795-805. DOI: 10.1016/j.det.2010.08.007. Review

[69] Pipkin C. Erosive diseases of the vulva. Dermatologic Clinics. 2010;**28**(4):737-751. DOI: 10.1016/j.det.2010.08.005. Lee KG. Papular acantholytic dyskeratosis of the vulva

[70] Werlinger KD, Cockerell CJ. Vulvar disease update. Advances in Dermatology. 2006;**22**:91-100

[71] Maldonado VA. Benign vulvar tumors. Best Practice & Research. Clinical Obstetrics & Gynaecology. 2014;**28**(7):1088-1097. DOI: 10.1016/j.bpobgyn.2014.07.014

[72] Stewart EG. Developments in vulvovaginal care. Current Opinion in Obstetrics & Gynecology. 2002;**14**(5):483-488

[73] Schlosser BJ, Mirowski GW. The diagnosis and treatment of vulvar and vaginal disorders. Dermatologic Therapy. 2010;**23**(5):435-437. DOI: 10.1111/j.1529-8019.2010.01347.x

[74] Jiang L, Wang JL, Zhu L. Summary of the national seminar on diagnosis and treatment of female vulvar-vaginal diseases. Zhonghua Fu Chan Ke Za Zhi. 2008;**43**(7):483-485

[75] Lang JH. Establishment and development the sub-specialty of vulvar-vaginal diseases. Zhonghua Fu Chan Ke Za Zhi. 2008;**43**(7):481-482

[76] Pichardo-Geisinger R. Atopic and contact dermatitis of the vulva. Obstetrics and Gynecology Clinics of North America. 2017;**44**(3):371-378. DOI: 10.1016/j.ogc.2017.05.003

[77] Edwards L. Dermatologic causes of vaginitis: A clinical review. Dermatologic Clinics. 2010;**28**(4):727-735. DOI: 10.1016/j.det.2010.07.004

[78] Akerman G, Dussour C, Haddad B, Paniel BJ, Rouzier R. Epidemiology of vulvar intra-epithelial neoplasias. Gynécologie, Obstétrique & Fertilité. 2007;**35**(12):1251-1256

[79] Soh HC, Russell P, Dalrymple C. Benign mixed tumour of the vulva. Pathology. 2005;**37**(5):389-392

[80] Perveen S. Benign tumours of the vulva. Journal of the College of Physicians and Surgeons–Pakistan. 2004;**14**(9):537-539

[81] Gupta R, Singh S, Nigam S, Khurana N. Benign vascular tumors of female genitaltract. International Journal of Gynecological Cancer. 2006;**16**(3):1195-1200

[82] Prabhu A, Gardella C. Common vaginal and vulvar disorders. The Medical Clinics of North America.

2015;**99**(3):553-574. DOI: 10.1016/j.mcna.2015.01.008

[83] Lai KW, Mercurio MG. Medical and surgical approaches to vulvar intraepithelial neoplasia. Dermatologic Therapy. 2010;**23**(5):477-484. DOI: 10.1111/j.1529-8019.2010.01351.x

[84] Shiozaki T, Tabata T, Toriyabe K, Motohashi T, Kondo E, Tanida K, et al. A case of usual (basaloid)-type vulvar intraepithelial neoplasia that failed to respond to imiquimod cream: Clinical implications. International Journal of Clinical Oncology. 2011;**16**(5):610-612. DOI: 10.1007/s10147-010-0180-4

Section 2

Therapeutic Depigmentation

Chapter 5

Depigmentation Therapies in Vitiligo

Sanjeev Mulekar, Madhulika Mhatre and Swapnil Mulekar

Abstract

Vitiligo is a chronic condition characterized by white patches on normal-appearing skin. It runs an unpredictable course. Main reason of stress in vitiligo patients is the presence of two colors on the skin surface. The aim of the treatment is to achieve normal skin color. Depigmentation is considered when repigmentation is not possible or the patient is willing to accept that repigmentation is not possible and opt for irreversible depigmentation. The only agent approved for depigmentation is monobenzyl ether of hydroquinone or monobenzone for patients with more than 50% of body surface area affected with vitiligo. The scope of this chapter is to describe modality of depigmentation and its risks and benefits.

Keywords: extensive vitiligo, vitiligo, depigmentation, MBEH

1. Introduction

Vitiligo is a skin condition characterized by loss of pigments on normal skin with a worldwide prevalence of 0.1–2%. Due to its cosmetic impact, vitiligo can impact the quality of life in children and adults. There are multiple therapies used for repigmentation beginning from topical corticosteroids, calcineurin inhibitors, and narrowband ultraviolet B (NB-UVB) to oral systemic medications and surgery. Even though a good number of patients may achieve successful repigmentation, there may be a few in whom the progression of vitiligo may affect extensive body surface areas making repigmentation an uphill task. The aim in such patients with extensive vitiligo (more than 50% body surface area) would be to achieve a uniform skin tone by depigmenting the remaining pigmented sites [1].

Depigmentation therapy is an accomplishable alternative therapy in patients who are extensively affected by vitiligo. It can be used in all skin types. Most readily used and available depigmenting agents are monobenzyl ether of hydroquinone (MBEH), 4-methoxyphenol, and phenol. Other therapies such as lasers and cryotherapy have also been used. The depigmentation process is a gradual one and can take anywhere between 1 and 3 years. In the author's experience, those who have undergone depigmentation are satisfied and happy with the therapeutic outcome if one achieves uniform color.

1.1 What the research says

The depigmentation approach is quite recent and is derived from the observations of unwanted depigmenting action of the phenol derivatives [2]. However, there are very few published studies on it. The aim of the researchers was to explain the possible mechanism of action for this class of compounds. Tyrosinase was the first suggested target. Also the potential of different phenol derivatives to act as an alternative substrate of the enzyme or as a competitive inhibitor was evaluated. Thus, it was hypothesized that this class of substances, or some of them, may be used for the treatment of skin disorders caused due to hyperpigmentation or melanocyte hyperproliferation. Further structural studies have indicated that the role of the position and type of substitutes in the phenolic ring allow the compound to be hydroxylated or oxidated by tyrosinase [3]. Considering phenol derivatives have a role in this process, hydroquinone was evaluated. Hydroquinone (HQ) belongs to the phenol/catechol class of chemical agents. Tyrosinase gets inhibited by HQ when interaction occurs with copper at the active site. This further decreases the amount of intracellular glutathione and induces the production of oxygen-reactive species. Thus, HQ acts as an alternative substrate, according to most part of phenol/catechol compounds, because it is similar to tyrosine. The enzyme can thus oxidize HQ without generating the pigment. The quinones produced are able to react with the sulfhydryl residues of the proteins, generating oxidative damage and affecting the cell growth. The depigmenting action is the result of the oxidative damage, involving both lipids and proteins of the cellular membranes. Functional studies have demonstrated that HQ and other phenolic compounds, such as tert-butylphenol, may even act through different mechanisms, including the oxidation of TRP1, and by interfering with RNA and DNA synthesis. HQ has been identified as the main depigmenting agent, whereas among the various phenolic derivatives, the monobenzyl ether of hydroquinone (MBEH) appeared as the more handful one. In this chapter, we will review and compare various established and potential depigmentation agents as well as emerging therapies that can be used in extensive and universal vitiligo.

2. Selecting the right candidate

Selection of an appropriate patient is of utmost importance in depigmentation therapy. The option of depigmentation should be made available to only those patients having extensive vitiligo. Detailed and thorough consultation sessions should be conducted with the patient and their families (preferably 2–3 sessions), explaining to them in detail that this therapeutic modality utilizes a potent depigmenting agent and should not be used for cosmetic purposes [2, 3]. They should be explained with all realistic expectations, treatment time frame, the cost involved, and side effects if any, and that once one particular type of treatment is done, they will not be a good candidate for any other type of treatment. Subjects with skin types (V and VI) with a disfiguring contrast between dark-pigmented skin and white vitiliginous areas, especially involving exposed areas (face or the hands), may be a candidate for depigmentation. Moreover, incomplete or trichrome repigmentation (e.g., when using UV light) may cause more disfigurement, thus making such individuals good candidates for depigmentation therapy. The patients should be informed that even after depigmentation, spontaneous repigmentation might occur in vitiligo lesions, warranting additional depigmenting cycles. Patients must be informed that these treatments lead to a definitive irreversible depigmentation. Younger patients with extensive involvement can be given an option of repigmentation instead of opting for depigmentation explaining that complete repigmentation may or may not be achieved. Depigmentation therapy should be avoided in children less than 12 years of age [4].

3. Topical therapies for depigmentation

3.1 Monobenzyl ether of hydroquinone (MBEH)

MBEH (monobenzone, p-benzyloxy-phenol) is the most common topical depigmenting agent used mainly because it is the only product approved by the United States Food and Drug Administration (USFDA) for depigmentation in vitiligo, if the affected body surface area is more than 50% [1]. It is a hydroquinone (HQ) derivative and was first introduced in 1930s. MBEH is the first-line agent for depigmentation therapy in vitiligo patients.

3.1.1 Mechanism of action

There are multiple pathways through which MBEH causes depigmentation [5]:

1. Reaction with tyrosinase enzyme during melanin synthesis leads to conversion of MBEH to quinones. The reactive quinone products formed bind with cysteine found in tyrosinase proteins (sulfhydryl (-SH) group) to form hapten-carrier compounds resulting in formation of neoantigens. These neoantigens stimulate a systemic, melanocyte destruction and an inflammatory reaction.

2. Another result of MBEH conversion by tyrosinase is production of reactive oxygen species (ROS). ROS leads to lysosomal degradation of melanosomes. Additionally, there is interference of the melanosome structure and membranes, following which the major histocompatibility complex (MHC) class I and II routes and initiation of melanocyte Ag-specific T-cell responses cause an increase in surface expression of melanosomal antigens.

3. ROS also contributes to an innate immune response due to the release of exosomes.

4. MBEH-exposed skin presents with rapid and persistent innate immune activation. It is quoted by Gupta et al. "that MBEH is a contact-sensitizer, inducer of a type IV delayed type hypersensitivity response against the quinone hapten. However, this only occurs if there is production of pro-inflammatory cytokines such as interleukin (IL)-1b and IL-18 by the Langerhans cells or keratinocytes" [6].

There have been reports that when MBEH therapy was combined with all-trans retinoic acid (ATRA), it enhanced depigmentation process and the melanocytotoxic effects via inhibition of the enzyme glutathione S-transferase in melanocytes. This could be a possible way to avoid contact dermatitis when using high concentrations of 40% MBEH. However, combination of ATRA-MBEH did not affect hair pigmentation in animal studies [7].

3.1.2 Administration of treatment

After the patient has been duly consulted and informed about all the possible outcomes and consequences of the treatment, the depigmentation therapy is initiated. Application of MBEH can be done by the patient at home. Initially, the exposed areas are treated. A test spot is advised over a normal pigmented skin (usually forearm) to assess the development of contact dermatitis. If there is no adverse reaction, the patient can continue with the application of the cream on the areas of top priority and then move in stages for low priority areas. To avoid contact dermatitis, different concentrations of MBEH can be used. MBEH can be diluted to 5% for use on the neck, 10% on the face, and 20% on the arms and legs. In patients who fail to respond to 20% MBEH over a course of 3 to 4 months, the concentration of MBEH can be increased to 30% and then further to 40%. Concentrations of 30 and 40% MBEH have been used primarily on the extremities, especially the elbows and knees. Concentrations greater than this are not recommended [8].

It takes anywhere between 4 and 12 months for gradual depigmentation [8]. It is to be noted that depigmentation is mostly irreversible and histologically associated with loss of melanosomes and melanocytes [1].

3.1.3 Precautions

Patients should always be informed and well instructed about certain precautions while using MBEH.

1. Application of MBEH at one site can lead to loss of pigment at distant body sites, i.e., application of MBEH to the arm may result in loss of pigment on the face [4]. Moreover, it can also reactivate a stable disease.

2. Application of MBEH to the eyelids is not advised [8] because of risk of ochronosis. It may lead to pigmentation of the conjunctiva if MBEH is applied on the eyelids.

3. Avoid skin-to-skin contact on a continuous basis with another person as it can cause a decrease in pigmentation at the site of contact in the other person.

4. The use of sunscreens with a high-sun protection factor (SPF) is essential. This also helps to prevent repigmentation as well as sunburn reactions [4].

5. Follicular repigmentation may occur spontaneously upon sun exposure [8]. This happens mainly because MBEH only destroys epidermal melanocytes keeping follicular melanocytes intact.

3.1.4 Side effects

Irritant contact dermatitis and common allergic reactions can develop [9]. In which event, application of MBEH is stopped, and open wet dressings are applied to the affected area along with topical steroids. Once the dermatitis has subsided, MBEH can be restarted at a lower concentration of 5% [8]. Other side effects include exogenous ochronosis [10], unmasking of telangiectasias and phlebectasias on the lower extremities [8], pruritus, xerosis, erythema, rash, edema, conjunctival melanosis, and distant depigmentation [4].

Risk of carcinogenesis with MBEH has not been reported but cannot be ruled out, and hence it is banned from the European Union since 2001 in cosmetics [11].

3.1.5 Combination therapy

All-trans retinoic acid (RA), which is a vitamin A derivative primarily employed in the treatment of acne, is shown to serve as a weak depigmenting agent when used for several weeks.

A combination or RA and MBEH induced significant depigmentation within 4–8 weeks. Nair et al. proposed that RA might enhance the skin penetration of depigmenting agents. Thus, RA increases the susceptibility of melanocytes to hydroquinone and 4-hydroxyanisole via the impairment of glutathione-dependent defense mechanisms of melanocytes and reducing melanogenesis activity in viable melanocytes [12–15].

3.2 Monomethyl ether of hydroquinone/4–0 methoxyphenol

This compound is a phenol derivative and is also known as p-hydroxyanisole (HA) or mequinol [1].

3.2.1 Mechanism of action

Mequinol acts in the similar way as MBEH acts. This compound usually acts via a dose-dependent response manner. It can be used as monotherapy or in conjunction with a Q-switched ruby laser.

3.2.2 Administration of treatment

The compound is used in a 20% concentration in an oil/water cream base. As with MBEH, cream is applied on an initial test patch to observe for any allergic reactions. If there are no reactions, the patient is advised to apply cream twice daily until complete depigmentation is observed [16]. The effectiveness of 4-MP has been correlated with the duration of the use of the cream; the longer the cream was used, better the results that were obtained [1].

A combination product of 2% 4-hydroxyanisole (mequinol) and 0.01% tretinoin was tested in a double-blind multicentric study and was found to significantly improve solar lentigines and related hyperpigmented lesions of the face and hands after a twice-daily application of up to 24 weeks [1].

3.2.3 Side effects

Side effects include mild burning or itching, irregular leukoderma, contact dermatitis, ochronosis, and risk of carcinogenesis cannot be ruled out [11]. Protection from sunlight is necessary or repigmentation risk is high [1, 11].

3.3 Phenol solution (88%)

Phenol is an inexpensive peeling agent having medium-depth capability and used for treatment of photodamage or rhytids. The toxicity of phenol toward melanocytes is well documented. Phenol has the ability to penetrate deeper into the tissue up to the upper reticular dermis.

3.3.1 Mechanism of action

Phenol is involved in melanogenesis, inducing coagulation of protein in the epidermis. The melanocytes lose their capacity to synthesize melanocytes normally. This property of phenol is different than that of MBEH and hydroquinone wherein they destroy the melanocytes [17]. Hence, 88% phenol can be used as therapeutic option to eliminate residual normally pigmented lesions in patients.

3.3.2 Administration of treatment

The area to be treated is cleaned with spirit/alcohol. Application of phenol is done with the help of a swab soaked with phenol until cutaneous frosting occurs. There might be a burning sensation experienced by the patient for approximately 60 seconds, which gradually decreases in intensity but can last from minutes to hours. In a case study reported by Zanini and Machado Filho, they reported the use of 88% phenol on a 62-year-old female patient. Post 2 sessions, with a gap of 45 days, total elimination of residual pigmentation was achieved [17].

3.3.3 Side effects

In general, 88% phenol does not produce any major complications when used in limited areas. However, some complications such as cardiotoxicity and other systemic toxicities have been reported in patients treated with medium and deep peeling over larger areas. Its cellular uptake is both rapid and passive because of its lipophilic character and signs of systemic toxicity develop soon after exposure. Cardiovascular shock, cardiac arrhythmias, and bradycardia, as well as metabolic acidosis, have been reported within 6 hours of skin-peeling procedures with phenol [17]. Other complications include non-esthetic scar formation, dyschromia, and development of herpetic eczema. However, the authors of this chapter have also noted a paradoxical response, wherein phenol application led to repigmentation of the skin!

4. Physical therapies for depigmentation

Depigmentation with topicals is effective; however, they come with their share of side effects and can take up to 10 months or more for completion of the process and rarely complete depigmentation may not be achieved. Depigmentation by physical means, i.e., by cryotherapy and lasers, can be done when rapid depigmentation is desired or when patients have not responded well to topicals or have had contact dermatitis or any side effects due to the same.

4.1 Cryotherapy

Cryotherapy is nothing but cold therapy or the use of low temperatures to treat a variety of tissue lesions. With cryotherapy, it is possible to achieve rapid and permanent depigmentation via irreversible tissue damage resulting from intracellular ice formation. Liquid nitrogen is used as a cryogen for clinical use. The degree of damage depends on the rate of cooling and minimum temperature achieved. Further, inflammation develops within 24 hours of the treatment, which contributes to destruction of lesions via immunologically mediated mechanisms. In areas of koebnerization, cryotherapy is more effective.

4.1.1 Procedure

Initially, spot testing by a single freeze-thaw cycle is done. Once the edema and erythema subside, patches are treated with cryotherapy 3–6 weeks later. Either CO_2 or liquid N_2 can be used. A 2-cm flat-topped and round cryoprobe is used at approximately 40 mm from the skin surface. The whole patch is frozen with a single freeze-thaw cycle from the periphery followed by forming successive rows inward.

Procedure should be terminated when a narrow (<1 mm) frost rim forms around the periphery of the cryoprobe. The rim can develop within 10–20 s by a cryogun connected to a container with barometric pressure above 80 kg/cm^2. For lesions around the orbits or uneven areas of the nose, cryoprobes having smaller diameters may be required. No more than one freeze-thaw cycle is advised per session. There have been cases reported which have used two freeze-thaw cycles [18]. Results are visible by the end of 4 weeks after the procedure.

Alternatively, a cryospray/cryopen or the traditional dip-stick method of application can be used following the same freeze-thaw cycle protocol.

4.1.2 Pros and cons

- Low cost and simple to perform.
- Does not require anesthesia.
- Minimal wound care with no dressing or antibiotics.
- Safe and efficacious.
- No scar formation if performed by an experienced dermatologist.
- It can be performed only on smaller areas.
- Multiple sittings may be required.
- If performed aggressively, it can lead to permanent scarring.

4.2 Laser therapy

Another faster method of depigmentation is the use of laser therapy. Lasers have been advocated more than MBEH and other bleaching agents due to their failure rate, as they have been proven to selectively destruct the melanocytes causing depigmentation. Further the risk of scar formation is minimized with laser therapies [16].

Mainly, the Q-switched ruby (QSR, 694 nm) and alexandrite (755 nm) lasers have been used in depigmentation. Both of these lasers operate in a similar manner in terms of mechanism of action. They induce photothermolysis of the pigmented lesions as they have wavelengths between 600 and 800 nm. These wavelengths are more readily and well absorbed by melanin. The frequency and pulse width is adjusted according to the skin type of the patient by a trained and experienced dermatologist. A maximum of 80 cm^2 area is treated per session.

Q-switched ruby	Q-switched alexandrite
• Selectively targets melanosomes and destroys melanocytes and keratinocytes • Works better on tanned skin • Fast and safe • Duration of treatment is short • Larger areas can be treated effectively • Reduced risk of scar formation	• Is efficacious in treating naturally occurring pigmented lesions as well as exogenous pigments • Safe, simple, and effective in treating recalcitrant pigmentation • Faster pulse frequency, hence rapid therapy • Higher wavelength so greater tissue penetration with improved results

Some other potential Q-switched lasers that can selectively destruct melanocytes include neodymium:yttrium aluminum garnet (Nd:YAG) laser (1064 nm) and the frequency-doubled Q-switched Nd:YAG laser (532 nm) [1]. In a study by Boen et al., Q-switched ruby laser (QSRL) 694 nm, Q-switched alexandrite laser (QSAL) 755 nm, and picosecond 755-nm alexandrite lasers provided the most significant pigment reduction when different recalcitrant pigmented areas of the body were treated by the abovementioned lasers over different areas in the same patient. In all the patients treated with this laser therapy, no adverse reactions apart from mild postprocedure erythema and crusting were noticed. The picosecond laser poses more advantages over the traditional Q-switch laser as it has increased photochemical action due to shorter pulse duration, requires lesser treatment sessions, and has reduced specific photothermal damage. This results in an increase in the safety profile of the laser and improves the effectiveness of this therapeutic modality [19, 24–26].

4.2.1 Points to ponder

- Procedure is slightly painful and may require local anesthesia.
- Treatment is expensive.
- Possibility of failure in removing pigmented patches even after several treatments because of Koebner's phenomenon.
- Patients with active vitiligo respond better to laser treatments compared to those with stable vitiligo. Hence, patients who are Koebner negative may often relapse [16].

5. Emerging therapies for depigmentation

5.1 Imatinib

Also known as imatinib mesylate, it is used to treat conditions like leukemia and gastrointestinal stromal tumors. It was observed that patients treated with imatinib were reported to develop generalized depigmentation as a side effect. Imatinib is a tyrosinase kinase inhibitor, thus inhibiting the activity of the enzyme, resulting in decreased pigmentation of the skin. The side effects of imatinib include fluid retention, periorbital edema, diarrhea, and myelosuppression. Some of the dermatological side effects include erythroderma, follicular mucinosis, and lichenoid eruption [27].

5.2 Imiquimod

Imiquimod is usually used for topical treatment of anogenital warts and basal cell carcinomas [20]. It is an imidazoquinoline and is an immune response modifier. It acts by stimulating the monocytes/macrophages and plasmacytoid dendritic cells in dermis and epidermis of the immune system to produce pro-inflammatory cytokines, mainly interferon α and other signals that activate T-cell-mediated response leading to apoptosis of tumor cells. Prolonged use of imiquimod has shown to result in depigmentation [1]. Imiquimod also stimulates CD8 cells to become cytotoxic and enhances antigen presentation [21]. Recently, it was reported that human melanocytes express toll-like receptor 7 (TLR7). When applied topically, imiquimod binds to TLR7 followed by stimulation of various cytokines, which induce the abovementioned T-lymphocytic response [22]. Imiquimod also has a direct action on melanocytes via apoptosis of melanocytes. This action is related to reduction of expression of Bcl-2 and/or an increase in the proapoptotic stimulus (cytotoxic T lymphocytes, natural cytotoxic T cells/killer cells, granzymes B, Fas, TNF, Bax, etc.) [23].

Thus, there is a strong possibility that imiquimod may cause elimination of melanocytes by direct influence on cells as well as inducing acquired immunity indirectly, which eventually induces vitiligo-like hypopigmented lesions [28]. Some common side effects include itching, pain, burning, erosions, erythema, and crusting.

5.3 Diphencyprone (DPCP)

DPCP is used traditionally as a treatment modality for alopecia areata. Depigmentation was found to be one of the side effects due to the use of DPCP. It has an immunomodulatory mechanism of action. As reported by Duhra and Foulds [12], in a case of alopecia totalis where topical DPCP was used, there a was marked reaction with erythema and edema on the forearm after 3 days, but the scalp manifested only slight macular erythema. The reaction on the forearm subsided after 2 weeks and was replaced by a depigmented patch over a period of 6 weeks. Upon incubating the affected skin with dopa followed by electron microscopy, an absence of melanosomes and melanocytes was revealed. It has been observed that vitiligo can develop even with DPCP concentrations as low as 0.0001% [12].

Some of the adverse effects include hyperpigmentation, regional lymphadenopathy, blistering, and eczematous reactions [20].

6. Limitations

The science of depigmentation is still not a perfected one and that does leave many questions unanswered. Further research in this arena can help shed light on these doubts:

1. Aspects that cannot be controlled
    a. Remote depigmentation.
    b. End result (color matching or same color).
    c. Hairs do not lose pigment (can give repigmentation especially follicular).
    d. Repigmentation during pregnancy (at times extensive).
    e. Resistance to MBEH.
2. Can patients with less than 50% involvement, willing to accept that no more repigmentation is possible, are candidates for depigmentation?
3. Whether depigmentation in children is a safe and viable alternative?

7. Conclusion

Vitiligo has a huge psychological impact and is also socially stigmatizing, particularly for patients with darker skin types in whom the contrast between the vitiliginous lesions and uninvolved skin can be especially apparent and disfiguring. In patients with widespread involvement covering more than 50% of their body and in cases where medical modalities including phototherapy have proved ineffective, depigmentation therapy should be considered. Patient selection, adequate counseling, and patient education are extremely important for a positive long-term outcome.

Author details

Sanjeev Mulekar*, Madhulika Mhatre and Swapnil Mulekar
Mulekar Vitiligo Clinic, Mumbai, India

*Address all correspondence to: mulekar@gmail.com

References

[1] Alghamdi KM, Kumar A. Depigmentation therapies for normal skin in vitiligo universalis. Journal of the European Academy of Dermatology and Venereology. 2011;**25**:749-757

[2] Nordlund JJ. Depigmentation for the treatment of extensive vitiligo. In: Hann SK, Nordlund JJ, editors. Vitiligo. Lucon: Blackwell Science; 2000. pp. 207-213

[3] Solano F, Briganti S, Picardo M, et al. Hypopigmenting agents: An updated review on biological, chemical and clinical aspects. Pigment Cell Research. 2006;**19**:550-571

[4] Drake LA, Dinehart SM, Farmer ER, Goltz RW, Graham GF, Hordinsky MK, et al. Guidelines of care for vitiligo. Journal of the American Academy of Dermatology. 1996;**35**:620-626

[5] Van doon Boorn JG, Melief CJ, Luiten RM. Monobenzone induced depigmentation: From enzymatic blockade to autoimmunity. Pigment Cell & Melanoma Research. 2011;**24**:673-679

[6] Gupta D, Kumari R, Thappa DM. Depigmentation therapies in vitiligo. Indian Journal of Dermatology, Venereology and Leprology. 2012;**78**:49-58

[7] Kasraee B, Fallahi MR, Ardekani GS, Doroudchi G, Omrani GR, Handjani S, et al. Retinoic acid synergistically enhances the melanocytotoxic and depigmenting effects of MBEH in black Guinea pigs skin. Experimental Dermatology. 2006;**15**:509-514

[8] Bolognia JL, Lapia BK, Somma S. Depigmentation therapy. Dermatologic Therapy. 2001;**14**:29-34

[9] Lyon CC, Beck MH. Contact hypersensitivity to monobenzyl ether of hydroquinone used to treat vitiligo. Contact Dermatitis. 1998;**39**:132-156

[10] Charlin R, Barcaui CB, Kac BK, Soares DB, Rabello Fonseca R, Azulay-Abulafia L. Hydroquinone induced exogenous ochronosis: A report of four cases and usefulness of dermoscopy. International Journal of Dermatology. 2008;**47**:19-23

[11] Radmanesh M. Depigmentation of the normally pigmented patches in universal vitiligo patients by cryotherapy. Journal of the European Academy of Dermatology and Venereology. 2000;**14**:149-152

[12] Duhra P, Foulds IS. Persistent vitiligo induced by diphencyprone. The British Journal of Dermatology. 1990;**123**:415-416

[13] Njoo M, Menke H, Pavel S, et al. N-acetylcysteine as a bleaching agent in the treatment of melasma. Journal of the European Academy of Dermatology and Venereology. 1997;**9**:86

[14] Nair X, Parab P, Suhr L, Tramposch KM. Combination of 4-hydroxy-anisole and all-trans retinoic acid produces synergistic skin depigmentation in swine. The Journal of Investigative Dermatology. 1993;**101**:145-149

[15] Kasraee B, Handjani F, Aslani FS. Enhancement of the depigmenting effect of hydroquinone and 4-hydroxyanisole by all-trans-retinoic acid (tretinoin): The impairment of glutathione-dependent cytoprotection? Dermatology. 2003;**206**:289-291

[16] Njoo MD, Vodegel RM, Westerhof W. Depigmentation therapy in vitiligo universalis with topical 4-methoxyphenol and the Q-switched ruby laser. Journal of the American Academy of Dermatology. 2000;**42**:760-769

[17] Zanini M. Depigmentation therapy for generalized vitiligo with topical 88%

phenol solution. Anais Brasileiros de Dermatologia. 2005;**80**:415-416

[18] Di Nuzzo S, Masotti A. Depigmentation therapy in vitiligo universalis with cryotherapy and 4-hydroxyanisole. Clinical and Experimental Dermatology. 2010;**35**:215-216

[19] Boen M, Vanaman Wilson MJ, Wu DC, Goldman MP. Laser depigmentation in extensive vitiligo. Dermatologic Surgery. 2018:1

[20] Halder RM, Taliaferro SJ. Vitiligo. In: Wolff K, Goldsmith LA, Katz SI, Gilchrest BA, Paller AS, Lefell DJ, editors. Fitzpatrick's Dermatology in General Medicine. 7th ed. Vol. 1. New York: McGraw Hill; 2008. p. 61622

[21] Zirvi TB, Costarelis G, Gelfand JM. Vitiligo-like hypopigmentation associated with imiquimod treatment of genital warts. Journal of the American Academy of Dermatology. 2005;**52**:715-716

[22] Kang HY, Park TJ, Jin SH. Imiquimod, a toll-like receptor 7 agonist, inhibits melanogenesis and proliferation of human melanocytes. The Journal of Investigative Dermatology. 2009;**129**:243-246

[23] Kim CH, Ahn JH, Kang SU, Hwang HS, Lee MH, Pyun JH, et al. Imiquimod induces apoptosis of human melanocytes. Archives of Dermatological Research. 2010;**302**:301-306

[24] Thissen M, Westerhof W. Laser treatment for further depigmentation in vitiligo. International Journal of Dermatology. 1997;**36**:3868

[25] Kim YJ, Chung BS, Choi KC. Depigmentation therapy with Q-switched ruby laser after tanning in vitiligo universalis. Dermatologic Surgery. 2001;**27**:969-970

[26] Rao J, Fitzpatrick RE. Use of the Q-switched 755 nm alexandrite laser to treat recalcitrant pigment after depigmentation therapy for vitiligo. Dermatologic Surgery. 2004;**30**:1043-1045

[27] Leong KW, Lee TC, Goh AS. Imatinib mesylate causes hypopigmentation in the skin. Cancer. 2004;**100**:2486-2487

[28] Senel E, Seckin D. Imiquimod-induced vitiligo-like depigmentation. Indian Journal of Dermatology, Venereology and Leprology. 2007;**73**:422-423

Chapter 6

On the Intricacies of Facial Hyperpigmentation and the Use of Herbal Ingredients as a Boon for Its Treatment: Cosmeceutical Significance, Current Challenges and Future Perspectives

Naima Parveen, Ayesha S. Ali and Sharique A. Ali

Abstract

Facial hyperpigmentation is the term used to express areas on irregular pigmentation in the skin. It appears as darkened patches on the face that make the facial skin look uneven. Facial hyperpigmentation is not physically debilitating but has been associated with enhanced psychosocial complications including anger, depression and frustration. These psychosocial burdens, in turn, have inference on quality of life and self-esteem. So, the treatment of facial hyperpigmentation seems to be a growing concern to the dermatologists today and they have been practising several treatment modalities including chemical peeling, laser therapy, dermabrasion, etc. But, those are found to be associated with various after-effects. Hence, the use of plants and its products is highly recommended as they are reported with either none or fewer after-effects. The present chapter draws attention to the forms of facial hyperpigmentation with their aetiologies and available treatment options for them with associated side effects. Furthermore, we have discussed about the other side of treatment with herbal ingredients which are safe and have less or no side effects. This chapter will be of value to the dermatologists who are searching for naturally derived ingredients for treating facial hyperpigmentation, in line with consumer expectations and preferences.

Keywords: hyperpigmentation, psychosocial, treatment modalities, etiology, herbal ingredients, novel agents

1. Introduction

Melanin is the natural polymer pigment responsible for imparting color to the skin, hair, and eyes as well as provides the photoprotection of the skin against ultraviolet radiation. It is produced inside the specialized organelles, melanosomes of melanocytes through a complex process called melanogenesis. Although melanin protects the skin from UVB radiation damage, its overproduction leads to the problem of hyperpigmentation and its related disorders. Post-inflammatory disorders, ephelides, solar lentigines, melasma, etc. are the common diseases of hyperpigmentation. Skin color imperfection due to hyperpigmentation spots on the face causes psychological problems in patients and takes them far from their social life. The public perceptions of tanned skin as being healthy and attractive merged with growing demand of treatment of facial hyperpigmentation provoke huge interest cosmeceutically as well as pharmaceutically [1–4].

Facial hyperpigmentation is a common and emergent concern to the dermatologists today. Treatment for facial hyperpigmentation seems to be difficult as there is no universally accepted treatment for it, and also the efficiency of known active agents is different. Majority of reports concerning the treatment of the disease consist of small series of patients. So, it becomes challenging to evaluate the efficacy of variety of therapy. Moreover, there are various options, but some of them come under growing scrutiny, emphasizing the research into pathogenesis and treatment. Sunscreen, chemical peeling, laser therapy, dermabrasion, topical treatment, cosmetic camouflages, etc. are the different treatment modalities used to treat facial hyperpigmentation. Though they are very effective and instant treatment for hyperpigmentation, its long-term exposure causes various side effects. Persistent erythema, swelling, pain, allergic reactions, herpes recurrence, acne, dyspigmentation, etc. are some of the various after effects associated with these treatment strategies [5–7].

In opposition to the state of affairs with these treatment options, we have the other side with herbal treatment which are nowadays attaining importance due to their low cost and ease of use and are believed to be free from risk of handling them as well as scarcely pollute the environment. Consequently, a dermatological formulation, including active ingredients of strictly natural origin, is designed by a variety of scientist to protect the skin from exogenous and endogenous harmful agents. There are many chemical reactions involving various enzymes that are engaged in melanogenesis. So, there is a wide range of targets or mechanisms against which to screen for skin pigmentation control agents. Active compounds isolated from different plants inhibit melanogenesis with no cytotoxicity by different mechanisms including inhibition of tyrosinase and other related protein expressions, inhibition of tyrosinase activity, inhibition of melanin dispersion and translocation, etc. [8–10].

Hence, the present chapter highlights the commonly occurring hyperpigmentary diseases of the face and their aetiologies. The available treatment options for hyperpigmentation along with the problems associated with them. As there is vast flora available on earth which has valuable medicinal properties, they are used for the treatment of many incurable diseases. Consequently, plants and its products are used for the treatment of hyperpigmentation through different mechanisms of action. Various studies on the use of plants for hyperpigmentation treatment have also been discussed in the present chapter.

2. Biosynthesis of melanin

Melanin is the end product of complex multistep transformation of amino acid, L-tyrosine. It is the polymorphous and multifunctional biopolymer represented by eumelanin (brown-black melanin), pheomelanin (brown-red melanin), and allomelanin (nitrogen-free melanin). This can be differentiated on the basis of chemical composition and monomer subunit structure of melanin. It has been found that there are four factors involved in melanin formation: (1) tyrosine as substrate, (2) tyrosinase with its coenzyme, (3) molecular oxygen, and (4) dihydroxyphenylalanine (DOPA). Tyrosine is converted into melanin by a series of enzymatic reaction [11–13].

Biosynthesis of melanin can be initiated from either the hydroxylation of L-phenylalanine to L-tyrosine or directly from L-tyrosine, which is then hydroxylated to L-dihydroxyphenylalanine (L-DOPA). In the next step, L-DOPA is oxidized to dopaquinone which is common to both eu- and pheomelanogenic pathways. Formation of eumelanin involves transformation of dopaquinone to leukodopachrome, followed by a series of oxidoreduction reactions. Dihydroxyindole (DHI) and DHI carboxylic acid (DHICA) are produced as intermediates, which undergo polymerization to form eumelanin. Pheomelanin synthesis also begins with dopaquinone; this is conjugated to cysteine or glutathione to yield cysteinyldopa and glutathionyldopa, for further transformation into pheomelanin. Mixed melanin contains both eu- and pheomelanin [12, 14–18].

3. Hyperpigmentary diseases of the face and their etiology

Melanocytes are responsible for the synthesis and distribution of melanin pigment, by the process of melanogenesis which involves different stages from embryonic development, melanin synthesis, to its transfer to neighboring keratinocytes. The importance of each of these stages and their mechanisms is evident in clinical defects in the form of hypopigmentation or hyperpigmentation. Exposure of the skin to UV radiation or other exo- and endogenous sources/allergen poses erythema, variation of vascular responses and immunosuppression, formation of inflammatory mediators, or overproduction of melanin which leads to pigmentary disorder, i.e. hyperpigmentation [19–21].

Facial hyperpigmentation is a common and growing concern to the dermatologists today. The difference in structure and function of the skin, as well as the influence of cultural practices, produces variable skin diseases of the face based on skin type. There are many skin conditions quite unique to person skin of color. Some of them are summarized here.

3.1 Postinflammatory hyperpigmentation

Postinflammatory hyperpigmentation (PIH) refers to the darkening of the skin that arises after cutaneous injury or inflammatory eruption. Hyperpigmentation results from the melanocyte's response to the cutaneous insult, which causes increased production of melanin. Acne lesions, scratches, insect bites, ingrown hairs, etc. are among such cutaneous insults. It has been found that patients of darker skin are more susceptible to this pigment alteration. Postinflammatory changes can occur both in the epidermis and dermis of the skin. In epidermal hyperpigmentation, there is an increase in melanin production and/or its transfer to keratinocytes. In dermal postinflammatory hyperpigmentation, a damaged basement membrane allows melanin to enter the dermis, which is then phagocytosed by dermal macrophages, called as melanophages. Macrophages may also migrate into the epidermis, phagocytose melanosomes, and then return to the dermis. Melanin within dermal melanophages may persist for years [22–25].

Physical examination of PIH includes small to large hyperpigmented macules and patches of variable size in any distribution. The time required for the normalization of dyspigmentation is unpredictable and depends on many factors including the patient's baseline skin tone, the type and intensity of the injury or inflammation, and the patient's sun exposure habits [22, 24].

3.2 Maturational dyschromia

It has been observed as darkening of facial skin tone, even outside of extensive sun exposure and sometimes termed as general uneven tone. Maturational dyschromia can be described as diffuse hyperpigmentation usually occurs on the lateral forehead and cheek bones. According to one of the survey-based studies, more than one third of black women have complaint of uneven skin tone. These alterations in skin tone are possibly due to chronic sun exposure over many years. Maturational dyschromia may be misdiagnosed as melasma, acanthosis nigricans, or postinflammatory hyperpigmentation [26].

3.3 Ephelides

Ephelides, or freckles, are caused by an increase in photoinduced melanogenesis and increase in transport of fully melanized melanosomes from melanocytes to keratinocytes. It occurs on sun-exposed area of the body, predominantly the face, dorsal side of hands, and trunk. They are 1–3 mm hyperpigmented macules that are round, oval, or irregular in shape. They might increase in number and distribution but can fade with aging. Ephelides are benign and there is no tendency of it to transform into malignant. Ephelides are benign and show no susceptibility for malignant transformation. Some ephelides represent as a subtype of solar lentigo [27, 28].

3.4 Lentigines

Lentigines are found more commonly in white subjects including African-Americans and American-Indians. Individuals of skin type I and III are more likely to develop solar lentigines. Solar lentigines result from a local propagation of basal melanocytes and a consequent increase in melanization, differing from freckles, which result from increased melanin production. Like ephelides, they also occur in sun-exposed areas, particularly the dorsal side of hands and forearms, face, upper back, and chest. Solar lentigines are 2–3 cm well circumscribed, round, oval, or irregularly shaped macules that differ in color from tan to dark brown [29, 30].

3.5 Melasma

Melasma is a common and well described form of hyperpigmentation that is seen most commonly on the face. It is a common disorder of hyperpigmentation affecting millions worldwide and at least 90% of those are females. It predominantly affects women with darker skin types, i.e. Fitzpatrick skin phototypes III and IV. It has also been referred to as chloasma or 'the mask of pregnancy' because the condition is often associated with pregnant women. There is recently no exact etiology, but multiple factors like ultraviolet radiation, hormonal alteration, genetic predisposition, and/or inflammation have all been involved. Physical examination of the disease includes light to dark-brown patches with irregular margins usually distributed symmetrically on the centrofacial, malar, and mandibular regions and can also be seen on the forearms [31].

On the basis of location of melanin, melasma can be differentiated into epidermal, dermal, mixed, and indeterminate types. In epidermal type, the pigment is brown, and borders are well defined, whereas in the dermal type pigment is gray brown, and borders are scantily defined. When there is melanin in both epidermis and dermis, mixed-type melasma occurs, and the term interdeterminate type may be used when it is not easy to classify even with the aid of Wood's light [32].

3.6 Lichen planus pigmentosus

Lichen planus pigmentosus is an unusual variant of lichen planus common in individual with skin types III and IV. It affects young to middle-aged adults generally those from India, Latin America, and the Middle East. Clinically, there are oval or irregular gray-brown to brown macules or patches with usually diffused and symmetrical pattern on sun-exposed areas, including the forehead, and neck, or intertriginous areas. Lesions are often symmetrical and can present in unilateral, linear fashion. The etiology for the disease is unknown, but immunological mechanisms associated with cellular immunity and exposure to ultraviolet light appear to be concerned [33, 34].

4. Treatment strategies for facial hyperpigmentation

Treatment for facial hyperpigmentation seems to be challenging as there is no universally accepted therapy for it, and also the efficacy of existing agents is different. Majority of reports regarding treatment consist of small series of patients, so it is difficult to evaluate the efficacy of a variety of therapies. Additionally, there are multiple options available, but some of them come under increasing scrutiny, underscoring the requirement of research into pathogenesis and treatment. On the whole, treatment includes removal of provoking factors, photoprotection, and active pigment reduction with either topical formulations or physical approaches [35, 36].

4.1 Sunscreen

Numerous evidence-based studies showed that light from both UV and visible spectrum can induce variation in pigmentation pattern of the skin. Both UVA and UVB cause increased melanin synthesis resulting in delayed tanning. Sun protection is found to be the most significant step which has to be taken to prevent and to cure hyperpigmentation. So, broad spectrum UVA and UVB protective sunscreen with SPF of at least 30 including a physical block (e.g. titanium dioxide and zinc oxide) should be recommended in order to protect the skin from hyperpigmentation [37, 38]. It has been observed that the use of broad spectrum sunscreen on the first day after skin resurfacing can decrease the incidence of postinflammatory hyperpigmentation after laser treatment [39].

4.2 Cosmetic camouflage

Cosmetic camouflage is the application of makeup including cream and powder to conceal color. Physical blocking opaque sunscreens also have camouflage facial hyperpigmentation and prevent photoinduced darkening. Many patients find that the use of makeup helps even out skin tone. Moreover cosmetic camouflage solves the psychological problems that a skin imperfection is sometimes able to irritate; it allows to rejuvenate its own beauty and to return to its own social life [40]. A single-centre clinical trial was conducted by Roberts et al. on females with mild to moderate facial hyperpigmentation to assess the efficacy of multifunctional facial primer. They found it very effective for immediate or long-term improvement of hyperpigmentation when used over a period of 12 weeks [41].

4.3 Chemical peel

Chemical peels can be used for the treatment of facial hyperpigmentation either alone or combined with other regimens. Most common chemicals used for peeling are trichloroacetic acid, phenol, lactic, glycolic acid, retinoid, etc. In this technique, a chemical solution is applied to the skin which makes it exfoliate and ultimately peel off; it means it damages the skin in a controlled manner. Finally the newer skin appears with no hyperpigmentary spots. After chemical peel, the skin becomes more sensitive to sun, so the use of sunscreen is recommended. Generally, there are three types of chemical peels based on the depth of the skin they exfoliate: superficial peel, medium peel, and deep peel. In superficial peel, mild acids like alpha hydroxy acids are used to exfoliate the skin. It only penetrates the outermost layer of the skin. Trichloroacetic acid or glycolic acids are used in medium peel to remove damaged skin; they reach to the middle and outer layer of the skin. On the other hand, deep peels fully penetrate the middle layer of the skin. Medium-depth peel should be highly recommended and performed with caution, and deep peels are not at all recommended because of the high risk of permanent pigmentary changes. Although chemical peeling may help in improving facial hyperpigmentation, they can also cause irritation which leads to dyspigmentation [42].

4.4 Dermabrasion

Dermabrasion is the non-chemical superficial removal of the upper skin with abrasive tool. Patients with resistant melasma, especially with well-known dermal components that are hard to treat, have been successfully treated with dermabrasion. Methods with the use of 16-mm diameter coarse grit diamond fraise are considered successful. Ninety seven percent of patients were found to have improvement, and only around 1% was found to develop hypertrophic scars or permanent hypopigmentation [43]. In most of the other cases, mild to moderate improvement has been shown with dermabrasion. Histopathologically, decreased melanization and regular distribution of melanosomes were commonly observed in biopsy samples of patients treated with dermabrasion [44].

4.5 Laser therapy

Laser and light therapy is a promising and effective treatment for a variety of hyperpigmentation conditions. In particular, longer wavelength is the most widely used laser because it can penetrate deeper and can target dermal pigments. Lasers and light sources should only be used by the experienced physician, and it should only be attempted after other modalities have been proven to be unsuccessful for a particular disorder. This treatment strategy however is quite challenging because of the high risk of damage to surrounding tissues that can lead to long-lasting and delayed postinflammatory hyperpigmentation. So, proper patient counseling with regard to side effects, and expectations should always be done prior to any laser therapy [45, 46].

4.6 Topical treatment

The majority of topical agents used are those that disrupt the enzymatic processes of pigment production within melanocytes. Different agents like hydroquinone, kojic acid, arbutin, retinoids, etc. have been used either alone or in combination with varying degree of efficacies. Kligman formulation having combination of hydroquinone, tretinoin, and hydrocortisone has been used in many skin lightening creams. Modified combination of Kligman formulation has also been successfully tested by various scientists during their studies, and now they have been practised in various lightening creams. But continuous applications of these agents have been found to have certain side effects. Hydroquinone is the gold standard for the treatment of facial hyperpigmentation and has been used for many years, but adverse reactions have been associated with hydroquinone, which include asymptomatic transient erythema, irritation, and exogenous ochronosis [47]. Kojic acid is a known sensitizer and can cause erythema and contact dermatitis. Similarly, arbutin at higher concentrations can cause paradoxical hyperpigmentation [48].

There are various national and international brands who are claiming that the skin will glow after a short period of time on topical application of their cream. They are claiming that their products are entirely safe as they are using herbal ingredients. But, it is not possible to make the skin glow and white in a short span of time without using harmful substances such as heavy metals. The Centre for Science and Environment (CSE) has reported that about half of the 73 national and international brands of popular cosmetics contain high levels of toxic heavy metals such as mercury, cadmium, etc. The CSE's Pollution Monitoring Lab had tested popular fairness creams and found 44% mercury in it. According to Sunita Narain, director general of CSE, 'Mercury is not supposed to be present in cosmetic products. Its mere presence in these products is completely illegal and unlawful [49]'.

5. Consequences of conventional treatment strategies

Although there are several modalities of treatment for facial hyperpigmentation available today including physical therapies or chemical agents, none of them are entirely satisfactory. Traditional topical agents like hydroquinone, kojic acid, arbutin, etc. are highly effective, but their long-term exposure causes several side effects. Persistent erythema, swelling, pain, allergic reactions, herpes recurrence, acne, dyspigmentation, etc. are some of the various after effects associated with treatment strategies like chemical peeling, dermabrasion, laser therapy, and cosmetic camouflage [50, 51].

There is a high risk of damage to the surrounding tissues when treated with laser therapy. During one of the clinical trials on woman patients, allergic reactions have been reported when treated with chemical peel using tretinoin. Patients exhibited itching, swelling, and erythema on their entire face [52]. Though the use of sunscreen with 50+ SPF may protect the skin from sun tan, its long-term use significantly decreases the cutaneous vitamin D production which is necessary for bone health and hence increases the risk of osteoporosis [53].

6. Natural herbal-based treatment for hyperpigmentation

Due to the consequences of conventional treatment modalities for skin hyperpigmentation, scientists and dermatologists are now looking for the treatment which will be safe and having very less or no side effects as well as do not contaminate the environment. Thus, the use of herbs and their ingredients for skin hyperpigmentation treatment is gaining interest as they are found to be safer, milder, and healthier than synthetic products. Dermatological formulation, including active compounds of strictly natural origin, is designed to protect the skin from hyperpigmentation. The aim of using natural ingredients is to reduce skin hyperpigmentation without causing undesirable hypopigmentation and irritation in the skin [10].

As there are many processes and enzymes involved in melanogenesis, there is a wide range of targets or mechanisms against which to screen for skin pigmentation control agents. Active compounds extracted from different plants inhibit melanogenesis without melanocyte toxicity by different mechanisms including inhibition of tyrosinase and other related protein expressions, inhibition of tyrosinase activity, inhibition of melanin dispersion, and translocation.

6.1 Inhibition of tyrosinase activity

As tyrosinase is the key enzyme of melanogenesis, inhibitors of this enzyme have caught the interest of dermatologists to prevent abnormal accumulation of melanin. There are various botanical agents that are acting through interfering in the pathway leading to melanin synthesis by inhibiting the activity of tyrosinase [54].

p-Coumaric acid extracted from the fresh leaves of *Panax ginseng* was used to inhibit the oxidation of L-tyrosine catalysed by mushroom tyrosinase [55]. Epicatechin gallate, gallocatechin gallate, and epigallocatechin gallate were the three major components isolated from green tea, and their efficacy of the inhibition of mushroom tyrosinase was assessed and found that green tea was the strongest inhibitor. Kinetic analysis revealed that these components inhibit tyrosinase via competitive inhibition [56]. Similarly, studies of Hridya et al. [57] and Hridya et al. [58] demonstrated that brazilein isolated from *Caesalpinia sappan* and santalin isolated from *Pterocarpus santalinus* have been found to reversibly inhibit tyrosinase in a mixed-type manner. Both the compounds inhibited tyrosinase activity dose dependently.

Recently, Kim et al. [59] have isolated five flavonoids, kushenol A, 8-prenylkaempferol, kushenol C, formononetin, and 8-prenylnaringenin, from *Sophora flavescens* to find out compounds with inhibitory activity towards tyrosinase. They have tested the ability of these flavonoids to block the conversion of L-tyrosine to L-DOPA by tyrosinase. Among the five compounds, kushenol A and 8-prenylkaempferol exhibited potent inhibitory activity which was further confirmed by molecular docking analysis.

6.2 Inhibition of tyrosinase and other related protein expressions

To develop treatment therapies for hyperpigmentation, many natural products have been tested which aimed at inhibiting production and expression of enzymes involved in rate-limiting steps of melanogenesis pathway including tyrosinase, tyrosinase-related protein-1 (TRP-1), and tyrosinase-related protein-2 (TRP-2).

Macelignan isolated from *Myristica fragrans* has shown inhibitory action on melanogenesis and significantly decreased the expression of tyrosinase, tyrosinase-related protein-1, and tyrosinase-related protein-2 expressions in melan-a murine melanocytes. Macelignan effectively inhibits melanin synthesis and thus could be used as a new skin whitening agent [60]. Panduratin A isolated from *Kaempferia pandurata* was also found to inhibit melanin biosynthesis. Through western blot analysis, panduratin A has shown decrease expression of tyrosinase, TRP-1, and TRP-2 proteins [61]. Similarly, curcumin suppressed the expression of melanogenesis-related protein expression such as tyrosinase, TRP-1, TRP-2, and MITF in alpha-melanocyte-stimulating hormone (MSH)-stimulated B16F10 cells [62].

Panax ginseng is a medicinal herb, which contains various ginsenoside with therapeutic effects. Lee et al. [63] isolated floralginsenoside (FGA), ginsenoside Rd. (GRd), and ginsenoside Re (GRe) from *Panax ginseng* berry. Among the three, floralginsenoside (FGA) was observed to impart more inhibitory effect on melanogenesis through decreased expression of microphthalmia-associated transcription factor in a dose-dependent manner. In addition to this, FGA also induced extracellular signal-regulated kinase phosphorylation level in melan-a cells. Peng et al. [64] evaluated the antimelanogenic and depigmenting activity of 10-hydroxy-2-decenoic acid (10-HDA) from royal jelly of *Apis mellifera*. They have reported that 10-hydroxy-2-decenoic acid (10-HDA) would reduce melanin biosynthesis through inhibiting the expression of tyrosinase, TRP-1, TRP-2, and MITF in B16F1 melanoma cells.

In a recent study, Ko et al. [65] investigated that n-hexane fraction of *Sageretia thea* downregulated melanogenesis through reduced expression of tyrosinase, TRP1, TRP2, and MITF. Bioactive compounds responsible for melanogenesis inhibition were identified through gas chromatography-mass spectrometry (GC-MS) analysis as methyl linoleate and methyl linolenate.

6.3 Inhibition of melanosome transfer to keratinocytes

Regulation of skin pigmentation depends on several processes. The transfer of melanosomes from melanocytes to keratinocytes is one of the major factors which play a crucial role in cutaneous pigmentation. Hence there are various treatment modalities developed to inhibit melanosome transfer in order to prevent hyperpigmentation.

Niacinamide, a derivative of vitamin B3, can be found in many foods including meat, milk, eggs, green vegetables, etc. Greatens et al. [66] found that niacinamide inhibits melanosome transfer to keratinocytes in cocultures of keratinocytes and melanocytes. They have assessed the effect of niacinamide on facial hyperpigmented spots through human clinical trials and observed the reduction of hyperpigmented lesion. Methylophiopogonanone B extracted from *Ophiopogon japonicus* also appeared to reduce melanosome transfer [67]. Similarly, centaureidin (5,7,3′-trihydroxy-3,6,4′-trimethoxyflavone) derived from *Achillea millefolium* also reduced melanosome transfer to keratinocytes. It was believed that centaureidin activates Rho which leads to melanocyte dendrite retraction without affecting melanogenic enzyme expression [68].

7. Conclusion

Hyperpigmentation is a common condition characterized by patches or spots on the skin. Pigment spots appear mainly on body parts that are exposed and hence are more commonly found on face. Facial hyperpigmentation is not only the problem concerned with pharmaceuticals and cosmeceutical sciences, but it is a problem that can pressurized the beauticians also to find out its treatment. Besides of being a disease, it is also associated with psychosocial complications. So, the appropriate treatment for hyperpigmentation is the need of the day. There are various treatment modalities available in medical sciences in order to treat hyperpigmentation, but many of them come under increasing scrutiny due to the side effects they impart on the patient skin. Herbal ingredients on the other hand are free from side effects and can hardly contaminate the environment. Hence, they are used for the treatment of facial hyperpigmentation. Many plants and their products have been used successfully to treat hyperpigmentation. But still, there are infinite numbers of plants which are yet to be characterized for their efficacy to treat hyperpigmentary problems of the face. Scientists all over the world would therefore try to evaluate more potent agents using various state-of the-art techniques that are highly effective and safe for the treatment of hyperpigmentation.

Acknowledgements

The authors extend their heartfelt gratitude to the secretary and principal of Saifia College of Science, Bhopal, India, for the encouragement.

Conflict of interest

The authors declare no conflict of interest.

Author details

Naima Parveen*, Ayesha S. Ali and Sharique A. Ali
Department of Biotechnology and Zoology, Saifia College of Science, Bhopal, India

*Address all correspondence to: naimaparveen@gmail.com

References

[1] Maddodi N, Jayanthy A, Setaluri V. Shining light on skin pigmentation: The darker and the brighter side of effects of UV radiation. Photochemistry and Photobiology. 2012;**88**:1075-1082

[2] Ali SA, Naaz I. Current challenges in understanding the story of skin pigmentation—Bridging the morpho-anatomical and functional aspects of mammalian melanocytes. In: Muscles Cells and Tissue. InTech Open Publishers; 2015. pp. 261-285

[3] Ali SA, Naaz I, Zaidi KU, et al. Recent updates in melanocyte function: The use of promising bioactive compounds for the treatment of hypopigmentary disorders. Mini Reviews in Medicinal Chemistry. 2017;**17**(9):785-798

[4] Vera Cruz G. The impact of face skin tone on perceived facial attractiveness: A study realized with an innovative methodology. The Journal of Social Psychology. 2018;**158**(5):580-590

[5] Briganti S, Camera E, Picardo M. Chemical and instrumental approaches to treat hyperpigmentation. Pigment Cell Research. 2003;**16**(2):101-110

[6] Tadokoro T, Bonté F, Archambault JC, Cauchard JH, Neveu M, Ozawa K, et al. Whitening efficacy of plant extracts including orchid extracts on Japanese female skin with melasma and lentigo senilis. The Journal of Dermatology. 2010;**37**(6):522-530

[7] Gunia-Krzyżak A, Popiol J, Marona H. Melanogenesis inhibitors: Strategies for searching for and evaluation of active compounds. Current Medicinal Chemistry. 2016;**23**(31):3548-3574

[8] Kanlayavattanakul M, Lourith N. Skin hyperpigmentation treatment using herbs: A review of clinical evidences. Journal of Cosmetic and Laser Therapy. 2017;**20**(2):123-131

[9] Ali SA. Recent advances in treatment of skin disorders using herbal products. Journal of Skin. 2017;**1**(1):6-7

[10] Kanlayavattanakul M, Lourith N. Plants and natural products for the treatment of skin hyperpigmentation—A review. Planta Medica. 2018;**84**(14):988-1006

[11] Harmon LE. Melanogenesis and pigmentary disturbances. Journal of the National Medical Association. 1964;**56**(6):501-504

[12] Ito S. The IFPCS presidential lecture: A chemist's view of melanogenesis. Pigment Cell Research. 2003;**16**:230-236

[13] Wakamatsu K, Murase T, Zucca FA, Zecca L, Ito S. Biosynthetic pathway to neuromelanin and its aging process. Pigment Cell & Melanoma Research. 2012;**25**:792-803

[14] Pawelek JM. After dopachrome? Pigment Cell Research. 1991;**4**:53-62

[15] Pathak MA. Functions of melanin and protection by melanin. In: Zeise L, Chedekel MR, Fitzpatrick TB, editors. Melanin: Its Role in Human Photoprotection. Overland Park: Valdemar Publishing Company; 1995. pp. 125-134

[16] Prota G. The chemistry of melanins and melanogenesis. Fortschritte der Chemie Organischer Naturstoffe. 1995;**64**:93-148

[17] Haake A, Holbrook K. The structure and development of skin. In: Freedberg IM, Eisen AZ, Wolff K, Austen KF, Goldsmith LA, Katz SI, Fitzpatrick TB, editors. Fitzpatrick's Dermatology in General Medicine. New York: McGraw-Hill; 1999. pp. 70-114

[18] Kim J, Cho SY, Kim SH, Cho D, Kim S, Park CW, et al. Effects of Korean

ginseng berry on skin antipigmentation and antiaging via FoxO3a activation. Journal of Ginseng Research. 2017;**41**(3):277-283

[19] Elmets CA, Young A. Sunscreens and photocarcinogenesis: An objective assessment. Photochemistry and Photobiology. 1996;**63**(4):435-440

[20] An SM, Koh JS, Boo YC. p-Coumaric acid not only inhibits human tyrosinase activity in vitro but also melanogenesis in cells exposed to UVB. Phytotherapy Research. 2010;**24**:1175-1180

[21] Ali SA, Choudhary RK, Naaz I, Ali AS. Understanding the challenges of melanogenesis: Key role of bioactive compounds in the treatment of hyperpigmentory disorders. Pigmentary Disorders. 2015;**2**(11):1-9

[22] Masu S, Seiji M. Pigmentary incontinence in fixed drug eruptions. Histologic and electron microscopic findings. Journal of the American Academy of Dermatology. 1983;**8**:525-532

[23] Pandya AG, Guevara IL. Disorders of hyperpigmentation. Dermatologic Clinics. 2000;**18**:91-98

[24] Bolognia JL, Jorizzo JL, Schaffer JV, et al., editors. Dermatology. 3rd ed. St Louis: Mosby; 2012

[25] Passeron T, Nouveau S, Duval C, Cardot-Leccia N, Piffaut V, Bourreau E, et al. Development and validation of a reproducible model for studying post-inflammatory hyperpigmentation. Pigment Cell & Melanoma Research. 2018;**31**(5):649-652. DOI: 10.1111/pcmr.12692

[26] Baumann L, Rodriguez D, Taylor SC, Wu J. Natural considerations for skin of color. Cutis. 2006; **78**(6 Suppl):2-19

[27] Rhodes AR, Albert LS, Barnhill RL, Weinstock MA. Sun-induced freckles in children and young adults. A correlation of clinical and histopathologic features. Cancer. 1991;**67**:1990-2001

[28] Bliss JM, Ford D, Swerdlow AJ, et al. Risk of cutaneous melanoma associated with pigmentation characteristics and freckling: Systematic overview of 10 case–control studies. The international melanoma analysis group (IMAGE). International Journal of Cancer. 1995;**62**:367-376

[29] Rhodes AR, Harrist TJ, Momtaz TK. The PUVA-induced pigmented macule: A lentiginous proliferation of large, sometimes cytologically atypical, melanocytes. Journal of the American Academy of Dermatology. 1983;**9**:47-58

[30] Cario-Andre M, Lepreux S, Pain C, Nizard C, Noblesse E, Taïeb A. Perilesional vs. lesional skin changes in senile lentigo. Journal of Cutaneous Pathology. 2004;**31**(6):441-447

[31] Sheth VM, Pandya AG. Melasma: A comprehensive update: Part I. Journal of the American Academy of Dermatology. 2011;**65**:689-697

[32] Khanna N, Rasool S. Facial melanoses: Indian perspective. Indian Journal of Dermatology, Venereology and Leprology. 2011;**77**:552-563

[33] Kanwar AJ, Dogra S, Handa S, et al. A study of 124 Indian patients with lichen planus pigmentosus. Clinical and Experimental Dermatology. 2003;**28**:481-485

[34] Mulinari-Brenner FA, Guilherme MR, Peretti MC, Werner B. Frontal fibrosing alopecia and lichen planus pigmentosus: Diagnosis and therapeutic challenge. Anais Brasileiros de Dermatologia. 2017;**92**(5 Suppl 1):79-81

[35] Perez-Bernal A, Munoz-Perez MA, Camacho F. Management of facial hyperpigmentation. American Journal of Clinical Dermatology. 2000;**1**:261-268

[36] Rigopoulos D, Gregoriou S, Katsambas A. Hyperpigmentation and melasma. Journal of Cosmetic Dermatology. 2007;**6**:195-202

[37] Pathak MA, Riley FC, Fitzpatrick TB. Melanogenesis in human skin following exposure to long-wave ultraviolet and visible light. The Journal of Investigative Dermatology. 1962;**39**:435-443

[38] Mahmoud BH, Hexsel CL, Hamzavi IH, Lim HW. Effects of visible light on the skin. Photochemistry and Photobiology. 2008;**84**:450-462

[39] Wanitphakdeedecha R, Phuardchantuk R, Manuskiatti W. The use of sunscreen starting on the first day after ablative fractional skin resurfacing. Journal of the European Academy of Dermatology and Venereology. 2014;**28**(11):1522-1528

[40] Sheth VM, Pandya AG. Melasma: A comprehensive update: Part II. Journal of the American Academy of Dermatology. 2011;**65**:699-714

[41] Roberts WE, Jiang LI, Herndon JH Jr. Facial primer provides immediate and long-term improvements in mild-to-moderate facial hyperpigmentation and fine lines associated with photoaging. Clinical, Cosmetic and Investigational Dermatology. 2015;**8**:471-477

[42] Cestari T, Adjadj L, Hux M, et al. Cost-effectiveness of a fixed combination of hydroquinone/tretinoin/fluocinolone cream compared with hydroquinone alone in the treatment of melasma. Journal of Drugs in Dermatology. 2007;**6**:153-160

[43] Kunachak S, Leelaudomlipi P, Wongwaisayawan S. Dermabrasion: A curative treatment for melasma. Aesthetic Plastic Surgery. 2001;**25**:114-117

[44] El-Domyati M, Hosam W, Abdel-Azim E, Abdel-Wahab H, Mohamed E. Microdermabrasion: A clinical, histometric, and histopathologic study. Journal of Cosmetic Dermatology. 2016;**15**(4):503-513

[45] Polder KD, Landau JM, Vergillis Akrnel IJ, Goldberg LH, Friedman PM, Bruce S. Laser eradication of pigmented lesions: A review. Dermatologic Surgery. 2011;**37**:572-595

[46] Negishi K, Akita H, Matsunaga Y. Prospective study of removing solar lentigines in Asians using a novel dual-wavelength and dual-pulse width picosecond laser. Lasers in Surgery and Medicine. 2018;**50**(8):851-858. DOI: 10.1002/lsm.22820

[47] Westerhof W, Kooyers TJ. Hydroquinone and its analogues in dermatology—A potential health risk. Journal of Cosmetic Dermatology. 2005;**4**:55-59

[48] Draelos ZD. Skin lightening preparations and the hydroquinone controversy. Dermatologic Therapy. 2007;**20**:308-313

[49] Narain S. Centre for Science and Environment Report. 2014

[50] Shamsaldeen O, Peterson JD, Goldman MP. The adverse events of deep fractional CO(2): A retrospective study of 490 treatments in 374 patients. Lasers in Surgery and Medicine. 2011;**43**(6):453-456

[51] Costa IMC, Damasceno PS, Costa MC, Gomes KGP. Review in peeling complications. Journal of Cosmetic Dermatology. 2017;**16**(3):319-326

[52] Magalhães GM, Rodrigues DF, Oliveira ER Júnior, Ferreira FAA. Tretinoin peeling: When a reaction is greater than expected. Anais Brasileiros de Dermatologia. 2017;**92**(2):291-292

[53] Libon F, Courtois J, Le Goff C, Lukas P, Fabregat-Cabello N, Seidel L, et al. Sunscreens block cutaneous

vitamin D production with only a minimal effect on circulating 25-hydroxyvitamin D. Archives of Osteoporosis. 2017;**12**(1):66

[54] Gillbro JM, Olsson MJ. The melanogenesis and mechanisms of skin-lightening agents—existing and new approaches. International Journal of Cosmetic Science. 2011;**33**:210-221

[55] Lim JY, Ishiguro K, Kubo I. Tyrosinase inhibitory p-coumaric acid from ginseng leaves. Phytotherapy Research. 1999;**13**:371-375

[56] No JK, Soung DY, Kim YJ, Shim KH, Jun YS, Rhee SH, et al. Inhibition of tyrosinase by green tea components. Life Sciences. 1999;**65**(21):PL241-PL246

[57] Hridya H, Amrita A, Sankari M, Doss CGP, Gopalakrishnan M, Gopalakrishnan C, et al. Inhibitory effect of brazilein on tyrosinase and melanin synthesis: Kinetics and in silico approach. International Journal of Biological Macromolecules. 2015;**81**:228-234

[58] Hridya H, Amrita A, Mohan S, Gopalakrishnan M, Dakshinamurthy TK, Doss GP, et al. Functionality study of santalin as tyrosinase inhibitor: A potential depigmentation agent. International Journal of Biological Macromolecules. 2016;**86**:383-389

[59] Kim JH, Cho IS, So YK, Kim HH, Kim YH. Kushenol A and 8-prenylkaempferol, tyrosinase inhibitors, derived from *Sophora flavescens*. Journal of Enzyme Inhibition and Medicinal Chemistry. 2018;**33**(1):1048-1054

[60] Cho Y, Kim KH, Shim JS, Hwang JK. Inhibitory effects of macelignan isolated from *Myristica fragrans* HOUTT. on melanin biosynthesis. Biological & Pharmaceutical Bulletin. 2008;**31**(5):986-989

[61] Lee CW, Kim HS, Kim HK, Kim JW, Yoon JH, Cho Y, et al. Inhibitory effect of panduratin A isolated from *Kaempferia pandurata* Roxb. on melanin biosynthesis. Phytotherapy Research. 2010;**24**(11):1600-1604

[62] Lee JH, Jang JY, Park C, Kim BW, Choi YH, Choi BT. Curcumin suppresses alpha-melanocyte stimulating hormone-stimulated melanogenesis in B16F10 cells. International Journal of Molecular Medicine. 2010;**26**(1):101-106

[63] Lee DY, Lee J, Jeong YT, Byun GH, Kim JH. Melanogenesis inhibition activity of floralginsenoside A from *Panax ginseng* berry. Journal of Ginseng Research. 2017;**41**(4):602-607

[64] Peng CC, Sun HT, Lin IP, Kuo PC, Li JC. The functional property of royal jelly 10-hydroxy-2-decenoic acid as a melanogenesis inhibitor. BMC Complementary and Alternative Medicine. 2017;**17**(1):392. DOI: 10.1186/s12906-017-1888-8

[65] Ko GA, Shrestha S, Kim Cho S. *Sageretia thea* fruit extracts rich in methyl linoleate and methyl linolenate downregulate melanogenesis via the Akt/GSK3β signaling pathway. Nutrition Research and Practice. 2018;**12**(1):3-12

[66] Greatens A, Hakozaki T, Koshoffer A, Epstein H, Schwemberger S, Babcock G, et al. Effective inhibition of melanosome transfer to keratinocytes by lectins and niacinamide is reversible. Experimental Dermatology. 2005;**14**(7):498-508

[67] Ito Y, Kanamaru A, Tada A. Effects of methylophiopogonanone B on melanosome transfer and dendrite retraction. Journal of Dermatological Science. 2006;**42**:68-70

[68] Ito Y, Kanamaru A, Tada A. Centaureidin promotes dendrite retraction of melanocytes by activating Rho. Biochimica et Biophysica Acta. 2006;**1760**:487-494